Highway to

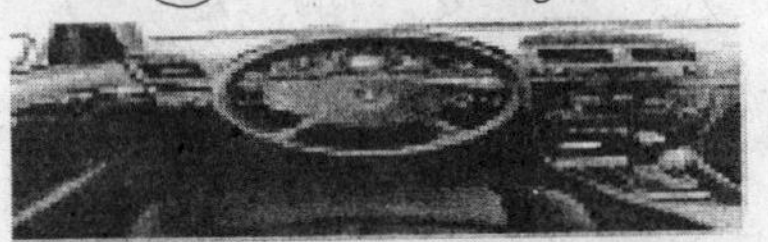

PLAB 2

Objective Structured Clinical Examination

Companion Volume

NHS Recruits
PLAB 2 Course Book

Highway to

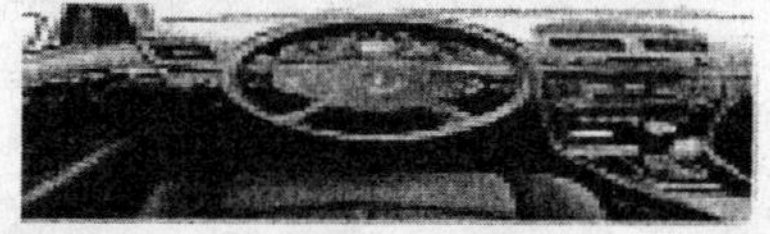

PLAB 2

Objective Structured Clinical Examination

A. UDDIN

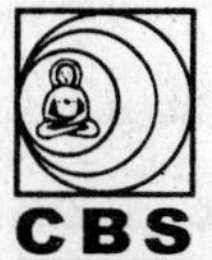

CBS PUBLISHERS & DISTRIBUTORS
NEW DELHI • BANGALORE

HIGHWAY to PLAB 2

First Edition : 2004

ISBN : 81-239-1047-9

Production Director : Vinod K. Jain

Published by :
Satish Kumar Jain for CBS Publishers & Distributors,
4596/1-A, 11 Darya Ganj, New Delhi - 110 002 (India)
E-mail : cbspubs@del3.vsnl.net.in
Website : http://www.cbspd.com

Branch Office :
Seema House, 2975, 17th Cross, K.R. Road,
Bansankari 2nd Stage, Bangalore - 560070
Fax : 080-6771680 • E-mail : cbsbng@vsnl.net

Printed at :
Asia Printograph, Shahdara, Delhi - 110032 (India)

Contents

to

---

my family
and colleagues

CLINICAL EXAMINATIONS

CARDIOVASCULAR SYSTEM

"Good morning,

I am Dr......................., SHO in this department.

Are you Mr......................?

Nice to meet you.

I need to examine your heart, is that all right?"

(Ask for chaperone and assure patient's privacy)

"Could you undress from your waist up?"

(Draw the curtains)

"I'll be waiting out, please call me when you are ready."

Position the patient at 45° with one pillow behind the back.

"Are you comfortable like that Mr..................?"

General

Mr.............. is not dyspnoeic.

Not in pain.

Hold his right hand and tell the examiner about

Hands

Cold or warm.

Dry or sweaty.

Nails

Cyanosis.

Clubbing.

Koilonychia.

Splinter haemorrhage.

Nicotine staining.

Palms

Palmer erythema.

Pallor (colour, creases).

Osler's node.

Cholestrol (tendon xanthomata, hardening of blood vessels).

Pulse

Radial

Rate.

Rhythm.

Compare volume simultaneously in both hands.

Collapsing.

Brachial

Volume.

Character

BP

Face

General (Down, Cushing, Turner, Marfans, ...).

Eyes

Corneal arcus.

Xanthelasma (check below eyes for cholestrol deposits).

Conjunctival pallor.

Icterus

Cheeks

Maler flush.

Lips

Caynosis.

Tongue

Central cyanosis ("Could you stick out your tongue please?").

Neck

JVP.

Carotid pulse

Volume.

Character.

Chest

Look

Chest deformity.

Scar.

Visible pulsation.

Feel

Localize the apex beat; its character.

Heaves (apical and parasternal)

Thrills

Auscultate

Apex S1 Intensity

"Could you roll over to your left side, take a breath in, take it right out and hold it?"

First diaphragm, then bell.

Pulmonery area (S2 intensity splits).

"Hold your breath on inspiration."

Aortic area (AS murmur).

Carotid

(Use bell, hold breath <5 secs)

Tricuspid area

"Could you sit up please, lean forward, take a breath in, take it right out and hold it?" (AR murmur)

Examine the back for

Basal crepitations.

Sacral oedema.

Abdomen

Liver enlargement.

Palpable kidneys.

Aortic and renal bruit.

Peripheral pulses

Femoral pulse

Radiofemoral delay (compare).

(Tell patient you are going to feel groin pulse)

Popliteal pulse.

Posterior tibial.

Dorsalis pedis.

Examine the optic fundi, fundoscopy.

Thank the patient.

** While auscultating the heart, describe what you hear carefully:

First heart sound and second heart sound are audible.

They are of normal intensity (muffled or not?)

Added sounds?

Clicks?

Murmurs?

CRANIAL NERVES II–VII

"Good morning Mr.....................

I am Dr. ...., senior house officer in the department of Medicine.

I am here to test your cranial nerves.

Cranial nerves are 12 in number and they supply the head and neck regions.

During the examination I have to touch your face, but at any time of the examination if you feel uncomfortable let me know.

Shall we proceed with the examination?"

I : Olfactory Nerve

"Could you smell that, sir, on this side?

What is it?" ("Excellent")

II: Optic Nerve

Visual acuity

Use either Yayegi chart or Snellen chart for near vision (the patient should wear his glasses).

"Cover your left eye sir.

Read the smallest print.

Thank you.

Again cover your right eye sir.

Read the smallest print.

Thank you."

Colour vision (is not essential)

Use Ishihara chart

(Causes: Congenital colour blindness 7%, age-related macular degeneration and optic nerve disease).

Visual field

(Sit directly opposite facing the patient)

Peripheral field

"Cover your left eye sir.

Just look there.

Please tell me as soon as you observe my waggling finger."

\/ Both upper and lower

/\ temporal and nasal fields.

Central field

(Use a read pin)

"Cover your left eye, sir, look straight here.

Do you see the read pin?

Good, keep looking at me, tell me when it disappears."

(It should be of similar size to your own blind spot)

Ophthalmoscopy (examination of the fundi)

Pupil

"Look straight ahead please, sir." (Look for size, equality and reflexes)."

Direct response to light.

Consensual (indirect) response to light.

Accommodation: "Look at my finger, sir, follow it in, in, in" (eyes adducting and pupils are constricting). (By this you can test for convergence as well)

III, IV and VI: Oculomotor, Trochlear and Abducent Nerves

Inspect the eyes at rest.

"Look at my finger, sir." (Position of the eye at rest, width of the palpebral fissures, *ptosis and squint*?)

Eye movements

"Please look at my finger and follow it wherever it goes. While I keep your head still with my hand, please tell me if you see double fingers."

(Check *for Nystagmus and double vision*)

V: Trigeminal Nerve

Sensory

"Close your eyes sir, say yes when I touch you (same, equal on both sides)."

Pin prick.

Corneal reflex: "Look to the opposite side sir (feel that alright), look towards me."

Motor

"Clinch your teeth" (feel temporalis and massetter muscles).

"Open your mouth wide, keep it open" (jaw jerk).

VII: Facial Nerve

Look at the face of the patient at rest for:

Asymmetry.

Involuntary movements.

"Raise your eyebrows. Wrinkle forehead.

Close your eyes tight, don't let me open them.

Show me your teeth.

Blow out your cheeks."

For sensory part—Shirmer's test (lacrimation) by blotting paper for 5 minutes.

It should wet >10 mm. Taste in anterior two-thirds of tongue.

VIII: Vestibulocochlear Nerve

Assess hearing acuity.

"Close your eyes, sir, repeat the numbers after me."

Tunning Fork:

Weber's test: "Do you hear that, sir, where?"

Renni's test: Air > Bone: "Which is louder, sir, that one (air) or that one (bone)."

IX and X: Glossopharyngeal and Vagus Nerve

Look at palate and uvula position at rest (in midline?)

Palatal movement: "Say Ahhh, sir, once more" (palate and uvula move at the midline symmetrically).

Perform gag reflex test and talk with the patient to see if there is any change in his/her voice.

XI: Accessory Nerve

"Do you mind slipping your top things off please?"

Observe the bulk of sternomastoid and trapezius muscles.

Power: "Shrug your shoulder up please, hold them there and don't let me push them down (trapezius).

Can you bend your head to left side please? Keep it there and don't let me push it to the right and vice versa (sternomastoid)."

XII: Hypoglossal Nerve

Look at the tongue at rest for:

Its position (midline).

Fibrillation.

Fasciculation.

Involuntary movements.

"Stick out your tongue please, sir" (midline)?

Wasted?

"Please stick your tongue on your cheek here, I'm going to press it."

Thank you very much for your co-operation Mr......................

RESPIRATORY SYSTEM

Introduce yourself.

"I need to examine your chest. Is that alright with you?"

Assure patient's privacy and ask for chaperone.

"Could you undress to your waist Mr ....?

And lie on the couch please.

Are you comfortable Mr....?"

General

Tell the examiner whether he is:

Dyspnoeic?

In pain?

Noises: Wheeze or strider.

Hand

"Hand can you give me your hand, Mr........."

Temperature.

Cyanosis.

Clubbing.

Nicotine staining.

Wasting of small muscles.

Wrist

Tenderness (pulmonary osteoarthopathy).

Pulse (rate, rhythm and volume).

Also count respiratory rate {N-12–16/min}

Flapping tremor

BP

Head

Eyes

Pallor,

Icterus,

Ptosis, constricted pupil? (Horner's syndrome)

Temporal recession (cachexia).

Lips and Tongue (central cyanosis).

Tonsils

Sniff- blocked **nasal airways**

Neck

Look

Use of accessory muscles.

Venous congestion.

JVP (raised JVP in pulmonary hypertension)

Feel

Crico-manubrium distance (4–8 cm) (< 4 cm in COPD).

Trachea (is it in midline): "I need to press on your trachea, it will be a little bit uncomfortable, is that Ok? Breathe in please."

For tracheal tug: the middle finger being pushed upwards against the tracheal rings during inspiration by upward movement of the chest wall.

Lymph nodes (cervical chain from front, supra-clavicular from behind).

Chest

Look

Shape.

Movement (symmetrical?).

Respiratory rate (16–18 cycle/minute), rib recession.

Scars /dilated veins.

Pigeon-, funnel-, or barrel-chest

Feel

"Have you got any pain in your chest?".

Tenderness / crepitus (subcutaneous / surgical emphysema).

Chest expansion: Apical/nipple level / lower chest (using thumbs).

Symmetry.

Apex beat / right ventricular heave.

Vocal fremitus ("say 99").

Percussion

"I need to tap on your chest, it won't hurt."

Listen

Same areas.

Air entry present, reduced or absent.

Character: Vesicular or bronchial.

Any added sounds: Wheeze.

Crepitation.

Vocal resonance ("say 99")

From back, examine the **back.**

Spine for tenderness.

Sacral oedema.

Examine the **abdomen.**

Examine the **legs** for swelling (pedal oedema).

Tell this examiner that you would like to check **sputum, PFR, temperature.**

Thank the patient

** In COPD, because of carbon dioxide retention, there will be:

Warm hands due to vasodilatation.

Pounding pulse.

LOWER LIMBS IN DIABETIC PATIENT

Introduce yourself.

Say: "I see that your blood sugar is a bit high.

I need to examine your legs.

Is that OK with you?"

You can ask for a chaperone.

"Could you take off your trousers but keep your pants please?

Could you walk a few steps (look for sensory ataxia – stamping **gait**)?

Could you lie down on the couch please?"

LOOK

Foot

Ulcer.

Gangrene.

Infection (fungal and bacterial).

Callus or cone (heel and head of **metatarsals**).

Small muscle wasting.

Pes cavus and claw toes.

Loss of hair.

Deformity.

Ankle

Deformity (Charcot joint).

Leg

Muscle wasting (measure).

Trophic waxy changes.

Knee

Deformity (Charcot joint).

Thigh

Injection site

Lipo-atrophy.

Lipo-hypertrophy.

Infection.

Quadriceps

Wasting (diabetic amyotrophy) (measure).

Feel

Pulses

Dorsalis pedis.

Posterior tibial.

Popletial.

Femoral.

Temperature.

Tenderness.

Neurological examination

Sensory examination

Joint position.

Vibration (128 Hz TF) (distal first).

Temperature.

Superficial pain.

Deep pain (disposable pin).

Light touch: "I'm going to touch you on the skin with this cotton. I want you to close your eyes and to say yes each time I touch you."

**Joint position, vibration, superficial pain and light touch are transmitted by dorsal column. Temperature and deep pain are transmitted by spinothalamic tract (lateral column).

Motor examination

Tone: Say "Just let your legs released sir, let them go loose and relax please."

Patella and ankle clonuses.

Power: "Please Mr....., relax and let your legs loose and floppy."

Flexors of hip: "Well Mr...., could you lift your legs straight up in the air, hold it there and keep it there as hard as you can, don't let me push it down" (L1, L2).

Extensors of hip: "Push the heel into the bed and don't let me lift the leg off the bed" (L5, S1).

Flexors of the knee: "Bend your knee and pull the heel in toward the bottom and don't let me extend" (S1).

Extensors of the knee: "Bend the knee up a bit, keep it bend up, hold the leg there and don't let me bend it" (L3, L4).

Dorsiflexion: "Pull your foot towards your face, cock it up, keep it up and hold it there, don't let me push them" (L4).

Plantar flexion: "Push your feet down, hold it down and keep it down, don't let me pull them" (S1, S2).

Toe flexors: "Cock them up, hold them up and keep them up, don't let me push them down" (S1).

Toe extensors: "Curl them down, keep them curled down, don't let me release them" (L5).

Reflexes

Ankle jerk (S1).

Knee jerk (L3–L4).

Plantar reflex (S1–S2).

If there is enough time, do heel-shin co-ordination test.

GASTROINTESTINAL SYSTEM

Introduce yourself, assure privacy and ask for chaperone.

"Could you lie down on the couch, please?

Are you comfortable?"

Hand: Nail (clubbing).

Palm: Palmer erythema.

Dupuytren's contracture.

Flapping tremor (30 seconds in cirrhosis).

BP.

Face: Pallor.

Cyanosis.

Jaundice (36 mmol/L bilirubin).

"Can you put out your tongue please?"

Dry or moist?

Furred or clear.

Foeter hepaticus.

Any ulcers in mouth? Infection?

Angular stomatitis?

False teeth?

Neck: Supraclavicular fossae.

Abdomen: Lie flat only on one pillow.

Look: Moves with respiration? (peritonitis)

Distension: Generalised.

Localized.

Skin: Hair distribution (cirrhosis).

Scar.

Spider navies.

Dilated vessels.

Visible pulsations.

Ask the patient to cough and look for any bulging (inguinal and umbilical hernia).

Palpation: "Is there anywhere that particularly sore?"

Superficial palpation for:

Tone, soft, easily compressed non tender.

If tense: Gurdening (peritoneal irritation).

If tense all time (rigidity in peritonitits).

Rebound tenderness?

Deep for any masses:

Any mass?

Site.

Size.

Shape.

Surface.

Consistency.

Attachment (superficial and deep).

Pulsation? (Pulsatile: Expansile or transmittable).

How you know the mass is deep or superficial?

"Please lift your head off the bed."

Organs

Liver: Normal is soft with smooth edge and not pulsatile

Its upper level is at 4th lower ICS (liver span?).

GB (rounding motion).

Spleen (smooth edge with tips).

Kidneys.

Pelvic organs: Bladder and uterus.

Pulsation.

Hernial orifices (lying and standing).

Percussion: Resonance.

Dullness.

Shifting dullness (only if the abdomen is distended).

Transmitting thrill.

Auscultation: Periumbilical for bowel sounds, if absent for 1 minute it suggests gastric outlet obstruction. Succution splash.

Auscultate for any bruit.

Examine the scrotum and rectum:

Scrotum: Deformity.

Assymetry.

Presence and position of both testicles.

Normal development?

Dartou's muscle contracted? (cold inflammation in the testis)

Palpate for tenderness:

Testicles.

Epidydimus.

Cords.

***Don't forget PR examination.

THYROID GLAND

Introduce yourself.

"I need to examine your neck gland to see if there is any problem.

Could you sit on this chair please?"

Expose.

General

Is the patient agitated?

Pulse:

Rate.

Rhythm.

Volume/compare.

Collapsing.

BP.

Start by inspecting the following

1. **Hands**

Nail changes.

Check for sweaty, hot, coarse or dry skin.

Ask the patient to outstretch both arms and fan fingers and look for fine tremor.

To check that, you can put a paper on the hands and watch for tremors.

Take pulses and mention about blood pressure.

2. **Face**

Check for any hair changes, excessive sweating.

Eye

Examine from front

For lid retraction and chemosis.

Ask the patient to follow finger up and down not too slowly. And look for *lid lag* (Von Graafe's sign). Ask the patient to follow finger up, down, right, left as it moves towards point. And look for ophthalmoplegia.

Ask the patient to tilt head down and to look upward, look for absence of forehead wrinkling (Joffroy's sign).

From back

Tilt the head back and support it with right hand and remove the hair with left hand. Look for *ptosis* (Nafzinger method of examination).

3. Neck

a. *Inspection*

For any mass (goitre) or lymph nodes.

Ask the patient to take a sip of water and look, and ask to protrude tongue and look for any thyroglossal cyst.

b. *Palpate*

(from behind)

Ask the patient for permission to stand behind and palpate for lymph nodes and the thyroid gland.

First palpate both lobes, then stabilize one lobe and palpate the other.

Ask the patient to take a sip of water and continue.

Then ask to breathe in deeply and palpate (check for stridor).

Check the position of trachea.

Percuss over the suprasternal notch.

Auscultate for bruit.

Lower limbs

Check reflexes of knee and ankle.

Look for pretibial myxoedema.

MINI-MENTAL STATE EXAMINATION

Greet

Introduce yourself.

Identify the patient.

"I need to ask you some questions which may sound strange to you Sir, but I need to check your memory."

Obtain verbal consent.

Orientation (10):

"What day of the week is it? (1)

What is the date today? Day, Month and Year? (3)

What is the season? (1)

Can you tell me what country are we in now? (1)

What is the name of this town? (1)

What is the street nearby? (1)

What floor of the building are we on? (1)

What is the name of this place?" (1)

Comprehension (3)

"I'm going to give you a piece of paper.

When I do, take the paper in your right hand (1).

Fold the paper in half with both hands (1) and put the paper down on your lap (1)".

Naming (2): (Agnosia; nominal agnosia)

Show a pen and ask what it is called? (1)

Show a wristwatch and ask what it is called? (1)

Repetition (1)

Say (once only) "I'm going to say something and I would like you to repeat it after me: No ifs, ands or buts".

Reading (1)

Say "Please read what is written here and do what it says".

Show a card with: CLOSE YOUR EYES written on it. "Now do what it says."

Writing (1)

Say "Write a complete sentence on this sheet of paper".

Drawing (1)

Say "Here is a drawing. Please copy the drawing".

All angles of the four-sided figure should be preserved.

Memory (6)

Say "I'm going to name three objects. After I have finished saying all three, I want you to repeat them (3).

Remember what they are because I'm going to ask you to name them again in a few minutes (3)".

e.g. "APPLE; TABLE; PENNY".

Calculation (5)

Say "Now I would like you to take 7 away from 100.

Now take 7 away from the number..., you get ?.. .. .

Now keep subtracting until I tell you stop".

Go on for 5 subtractions.

"What were the three objects I asked you to remember a little while ago?" (3)

Interepreting the score: **A score 28–30 does not support the diagnosis of dementia. A score 25–27 suggests dementia but consider also acute confusional state and depression. ~13% of over 75s in the general population have scores <25.**

PRIMARY AND SECONDARY SURVEY

First, you have to stabilize the neck if there is any risk of neck injury.

Primary survey

"Hello, how are you?

Would you please open your mouth and put out your tongue?"

Check airway, if it is clear.

If not, remove any obstructions, such as blood, teeth, and foreign bodies.

Inspect respiratory rate, bilateral chest movement.

Then auscultate to check for air entry on both sides.

If there is no respiration intubate and ventilate.

If respiration is compromised, put oxygen mask.

If there is tension pneumothorax, insert a wide bore cannula in second intercostals space at mid calvicular line.

Check pulse pressure and blood pressure.

If pulse is absent then consider the patient is arrested and treat accordingly. If in shock, start shock treatment.

Determine level of consciousness according to GCS, or AVPU.

GCS

a. *Best motor response:*

Obeys commands (6).

Localizes pain (5).

Withdraws or pulls limb away to painful stimulus (4).

Flexor response to pain "decorticate posture" (3).

Extensor response to pain "decerebrate posture" (2).

No response to pain (1).

b. *Best verbal response:*

Normally oriented (5).

Disoriented (4).

Inappropriate speech (3).

Incomprehensive sounds (2).

None (1).

c. *Eye opening:*

Spontaneous eye opening (4).

Eye opening to voice (3).

Eye opening to pain (2).

None (1).

N.B: Response to pain is best tested by pressure on supraorbital ridge.

AVPU: Alert, response to vocal stimulus, response to pain, unresponsiveness.

Exposure to check for further injuries,
and covering the patient to avoid hypothermia.

**Ask the patient if he/she feels any pain (assess verbal response), ask him/her to raise hand and to squeeze your fingers (motor) and look for eye opening.

Secondary survey

1. Head

Signs of injury as bruising, laceration, bony deformity, depressed skull fracture.

a. *Eyes*

Any foreign bodies, redness, perforation, size of pupil. Papillary reflexes, corneal reflexes, bruises around the eye (suggestive of anterior cranial fossa fracture).

b. *Nose*

Blood, discharge (bright red discharge suggestive of rhinorrhoea).

c. *Ear*

Blood discharge (let blood discharge on sheet, and look for double ring: mixed blood and CSF).

Bruises over mastoid (consider middle cranial fossa fracture).

d. *Mouth*

Check stability of maxilla and mandible.

Check for airway, any unstable false teeth or foreign body.

2. *Neck*

Check for subcutaneous emphysema, cervical spinous processes, venous dilatation, tracheal deviation.

3. *Chest*

Inspect respiratory movement, check for any penetrating or sucking injury.

Paradoxical movement of flail chest.

Palpate for tenderness, crepitus or rib fracture.

Percuss and auscultate checking for heamo/pneumothorax.

4. *Heart*

Auscultate for heart sounds.

5. *Abdomen*

Inspect for injury or echymosis, laceration, distension.

Palpate for tenderness, guarding.

Auscultate for bowel sounds.

Do digital rectal examination, check sphincter tone, and prostate.

6. *Diagnostic peritoneal lavage*

If in doubt, below umbilicus, put drip of 1 L N/S and aspirate.

7. Pelvis

Compressed and distracted manually to check for stability or pain, examine penis for blood drops (if present, do not catheterize).

8. Extremities

Inspect for bruises, laceration, or deformity.

Palpate for tenderness and stability.

Check pulses, sensory exam, reflexes, motor exam and muscle tone.

X-ray of spine (cervical), CXR, pelvic x-ray, blood for hematocrit, grouping and cross match, electrolytes, urea, glucose and ABGs. Do ECG.

EXAMINATION OF THE HANDS

Introduction.

Ask patient to expose both lower arms and forearms, hand resting, in comfortable position.

LOOK

Dorsal

Nails

Vasculitic and psoriatic changes.

Nail fold capillary (dilated or not).

Skin

Psoriatic changes.

Sclcroderma skin changes.

Blotchy erythema (dermatomyositis and SLE).

Vasculitic lesions occur on the extensor surfaces of the small joints (dermatomyositis).

Small muscle wasting.

Look for the presence and distribution of any joint swelling.

Deformity

Boutonniere's deformity.

Swan neck deformity.

Z deformity.

Ulnar deviation frequently at MCPs.

Subluxation of fingers at metacarpal heads.
Subluxation of the carpal bones of the radius.
Scar of previous surgery.
MCP, observe the gutters between MCP joints.
"Could you turn your hands over please *(palms)*?"
Palmer erythema in RA.
Muscle bulk (thenar and hypothenar).

FEEL

Dorsum of hands

Temperature
Mid-forearm – Wrist.
Mid-forearm – MCP.
Mid-forearm – PIP.

Tenderness
PIP.
MCP.
Wrist.

Swelling, e.g. effusion, synovial thickening or bony enlargement.
Is the joint actively inflamed?.
Wrist: For swelling, bony enlargement.
Bimanual palpation of MCP by index fingers for effusion rubbery.

Bimanually palpate PIP for effusion.

Firm pressure along PIP (rubbery synovial thickening typical in active sinusitis).

Firm bony enlargement (Heberdon's and Bouchard nodes).

Palmer Savill pinch test.

Feel the elbow for subcutaneous nodules (inspect for bursitis, psoriatic skin changes and gout tophi).

MOVEMENTS

"Turn your hands over please.

Make a full fist please and open it (flexion).

Could you stretch out your fingers (extension)?" (In RA extensor tendon rupture, finger drop.)

If the patient can make a fist, there is no need to test for the individual movement of the joints of the fingers.

If not:

Passive movements:

Flex and extend DIP, If they were restricted (contracutre).

Flex and extend PIP.

Flex and extend MCP.

If the above three were normal.

It's flexor tendon sheath.

So, feel the swelling nodularities and tenderness along the line of the flexor tendon sheath beneath the palmer face.

Flex and extend the individual fingers while resting your other fingers overlying that flexor tendon sheath to feel crepitus and movement with tension.

Thumb

"Could you bring your thumb right across the base of your finger?"

Attempt full flexion and full extension (passive).

Wrist

Prayer's test.

FUNCTION OF THE HAND

Grip

"Grip my hand firm as tight as possible."

Change object and position.

"Grip my finger (one finger) as tight as you can."

Pinch

Pulp pinch

"Pinch your index and thumb together, prevent me from pulling my fingers through."

Finger *tip* pinch (same).

Yayokee pinch (adductor of the thumb).

Hitch hiker (extensor polices longus).

Wrist

Flexion and extension power.

"Push down on my hand."

Cock back.

Ask the patient to undo a button or write.

NERVES

Carpal tunnel syndrome.

Tunnel sign (tap).

Phallen's sign (30 seconds).

Examine the sensory dermatomes.

Examine median, ulnar and radial nerves.

EXAMINATION OF HIP

Introduction.

Permission / chaperone.

Exposure (ideally expose the joint above and below, i.e. spine and knee).

Look

The patient in standing position

***Skin:* Previous operation scars infected sinuses.**

***Muscle*: Wasting – quadriceps, gluteal.**

Measure mid-thigh circumference.

Deformity

Adduction deformity.

External rotation deformity.

From back

Scoliosis.

Pelvic tilt.

Trendelenburg test (weakness of the abductor muscles).

Gait

Short leg gait (in destructive bone disease or CDH).

Antalgic gait (infection or arthritis).

Trendelenburg gait (lateral curving of the body).

Put the patient in supine position and inspect for:

Skin scar.

Muscle wasting.

Posture of the limb.

Deformity.

Feel

In supine position:

Bony points (measure and compare ASIS—GT distance).

Tenderness: Ask for pain before touching the patient (feel for pain at mid-inguinal point just beneath the femoral artery pulsation).

Measure leg length.

Apparent leg length (from xiphoid process to medial maleolus, legs parallel with patient lying supine due to fixed deformity).

True leg length (from ASIS to medial maleolus, legs should be in comparable position).

Movement

Position the patient, centre the pelvis.

Passive movements

Flexion (one hand stabilizing iliac crest, flexion 0°–120°).

Abduction 40° (stabilize the contralateral iliac crest.)

Adduction 30° (stabilize the contralateral iliac crest.)

Internal rotation 25° and external rotation 45° with the hip flexed at 90°.

Thomas's test (to unmask a flexion deformity of the hip concealed by presence of compensatory lumbar lordosis).

EXAMINATION OF THE BACK

Introduce / permission / privacy.

Exposure.

Look

From behind at standing position for:

Scoliosis.

Skin lesions (psoriasis or neurofibromatosis).

Muscle wasting.

From side, look for : lumbar lordosis, dorsal kyphosis, cervical lordosis.

Move

"Touch your feet.

Bend backwards."

Lateral flexion.

Schober test (15 cm).

Sitting: Move—lateral flexion.

Feel

Tenderness: "Could you lie on your tummy please Mr ...., do you feel pain anywhere in your back?"

Feel for tenderness in : Spines.

Interspinous ligaments.

Paraspinal muscles.

Sacrum.

Sacro-iliac joints.

Femoral stretch test.

Supine: SLRT (Bragaard test, Lasegue's Sign and Baw string sign).

Sitting: Flip test (malingering test).

KNEE EXAMINATION

Introduction.

"I'm going to examine your knee, please undress your bottom half to your underwear, and stand up for me.

Inspection

With the patient erect, then supine:

For limb alignment, bony contour, erythema, swelling, muscles wasting, and any genu valgus or varus.

Measures

Muscle girth at 10 cm above patella (both sides).

Palpation

With knee extended, palpate soft tissue, collateral ligaments for tenderness and temperature with dorsum of your hand.

With knee flexed, palpate along the joint line anterior and posterior for tenderness.

Movement

With patient supine, put your left hand on the knee to detect crepitation; ask the patient to fully flex knee and then to extend it.

With patient in prone position, thigh supported on the couch and legs projecting from couch.

Observe level of heels (test minor limitation of extension).

Tests

1. Massage test.
2. Patellar tap.
3. Patellar apprehension test.
4. Anterior and posterior draw test.
5. Lachman test.
6. Collateral ligament test.
7. Pivot shift test.
8. McMurray test.

SHOULDER EXAMINATION

Introduction.

"I'm going to examine your shoulder, if you don't mind expose your top half, please."

Inspection

Inspect the shoulder from the front, side and back for deformity, swelling, muscle wasting, and skin lesion.

Palpation

Swelling, tenderness in anterior aspect, bicipital groove, tip of shoulder, subacromial space and sterno-clavicular joint.

Movement

Ask the patient to place the palms at the base of neck with elbows pointing laterally.

Then put arms down and reach between shoulder blades with dorsum of hands.

Ask the patient to flex elbow to 90° and to do external and internal rotation of shoulder joint.

INTERMITTENT CLAUDICATION

"Good morning, I am Dr ...., SHO in this department.

I understand you have pain on walking that is why I need to examine your legs to find if there is any problem.

Is that alright?"

Assure the patient's privacy and ask for chaperone.

"Can you take off your trousers please and lie on the couch?"

Look at both feet and compare

Colour (pregangrene blackness).

Hair loss.

Missing toes, nail infection.

Muscle bulk.

Ulcers: Describe size edge base if it is arterial painful and punched out or venous painless.

Varicose veins.

Scars from previous operation in groin, and medial aspect of the thigh.

Gangrene.

Feel

Capillary filling (if abnormal Burger test).

Temperature (start from the feet upwards).

Pulses

Femoral.

Popliteal.

Posterior tibial.

Dorsalis pedis.

Palpate any varicosities (thrombophlebitis).

If the history is typical with I.C. and pedal pulses were present ask the patient to walk for few minutes and re-examine.

Burger test.

Auscultate aorta.

Femoral arteries.

I would examine the limb neurologically.

**Ulcer*: Site, size, edge, base, discharge (watery, bloody, pus) and colour.

Examine the LNs as well.

Types of ulcers:

Rolling or everted (malignancy).

Eroded (actively progressing).

Punched out (neurological or bed sore).

Slopping (healing ulcer).

Investigation

1. Blood tests: FBC, U and E, ESR, lipid profile, syphilis serology.
2. Ankle brachial pressure index: it is normally around 1, in intermittent claudication: 0.9-0.6.
3. Arteriography.

Management

1. Conservative: Stop smoking, loose weight; treat DM, hypertension, and hyperlipidaemia.
2. Angioplasty and arterial reconstruction.
3. Sympathectomy.

PROCEDURES

RECTAL EXAMINATION (PR)

Greet, introduce yourself and identify the patient.

Explain the procedure and its purpose:

Say, "Due to nature of your complain, I need to examine your back passage using my finger to see whether there is any problem and I'm going to feel your prostate also. It may be uncomfortable but shouldn't be painful. Please let me know if you have any pain."

Obtain verbal consent ("Is that OK?")

Ensure privacy and ask for chaperone.

Check the procedure's *requirements:*

A pair of gloves.

KY jelly.

A good source of light.

Ask the patient to undress from the waist below.

Position the patient (left lateral position)

"Lie on the left side, bringing the buttocks to the edge of the couch and drawing the knees up to the chest".

Ask "Are you comfortable?"

Put on the gloves.

Start the examinations

Before touching the patient, ask if s/he feels pain?

If there was any pain, consider using a LA.

If still painful, consider doing PR under GA.

Lift up the right buttock and look for:

Ulcer.

Discharge.

External haemorrhoids.

Fistula.

Fissure.

Skin tag.

Ask the patient to strain down, note for any extrusion of skin or mucosa through the anus.

Lubricate your right index finger.

Tell the patient that you are going to introduce your finger, ask him to breathe in and out and relax.

"Take easy breath please". Proceed slowly and note any tenderness or spasms as the finger passes through the anal sphincter.

Ask the patient to squeeeze or bear down his sphincter on your finger again to assess the sphincter power and tone.

Feel for any masses (soft, hard, smooth, fixed).

Note any surrounding lumps or nodularity within the anal canal.

Feel the hollow of sacrum and coccyx.

Turn the finger to the right side and feel for any caecal or appendical mass.

Turn the hand anti-clockwise, feel the left side of pelvis, and feel sigmoid colon.

Turn finger forward to feel prostate lobes.

Median groove.

Lump

Consistency.

Surface.

Upper edge (position of the pouch of Douglas for tenderness).

Further rotate the hand to examine the right side and ask the patient to strain down (any masses in rectum).

Withdraw your finger and look for blood, pus and mucous on your finger.

Test for occult blood (Guaiac test).

Give the patient a tissue to wipe himself.

Thank the patient for his co-operation.

Ask him to get dressed.

"I will come and explain the finding to you once you are dressed."

VAGINAL EXAMINATION (PV)

Greet, introduce yourself and identify the patient.

Explain the procedure and its purpose:

"I need to examine your front passage by finger to see if there is any problem, it may be a bit uncomfortable but it shouldn't be painful. Please let me know if you have any pain".

Obtain a verbal consent. ("Is it OK?")

A chaperone and ensure her privacy, give her a sheet to cover her waist.

Check the *procedure's requirements:*

A pair of gloves.

KY jelly.

A good source of light.

Tell the patient to empty her bladder and ask her to undress from waist down and position herself on her back to put her heel together and drop back her knees.

Put on the gloves.

Start the examination.

Separate the labia and look at the vulva for any:

- Discharge.
- Ulcer.
- Rash.

Inspect the vaginal wall and ask the patient to cough (for urinary incontinence) and to bear down (for prolapse).

Lubricate the index and middle finger of the right hand.

Before touching the patient ask her if she feels pain?

Tell the patient that you will introduce your finger.

Insert your fingers while labia apart,

Palpate vaginal walls (anterior, posterior, lateral fornices)

Obliterated and pouch of Douglas for:

Masses.

Cysts.

Foreign bodies.

Palpate the cervix and find out its

Consistency.

Irregularities (dilated or not?)

Move your fingers to note any tenderness (cervical excitation).

Do bimanual examination of the uterus, note for its:

Size.

Position (anteroverted or retroverted).

Surface.

Consistency.

Mobility.

Tenderness.

Examine the lateral fornices (adnexae) of uterus for:

Tenderness.

Swelling of Fallopian tubes or ovaries.

Examine the posterior fornix for uterosacral ligament (scarred or shortened in women with endometriosis).

Withdraw your fingers.

Give the patient a tissue to wipe herself.

Thank her for her co-operation.

Suggest speculum examination.

CERVICAL SMEAR

Greet, introduce yourself and identify the patient.

Explain the procedure and its purpose.

"I need to insert this instrument what we call speculum, into your front passage, to take a smear from the neck of your womb."

(Make sure that she is not menstruating, she didn't use sperm gel or lubricant gel in the previous 24 hours.)

Obtain a verbal consent.

Ensure her privacy and ask for chaperone.

Check the procedure *requirements:*

Cuscos speculum.

A good source of light.

A pair of sterile gloves.

Wooden spatula.

A slide.

Fixater.

A pencil.

Ask the patient to empty her bladder and get undressed from waist downwards behind the curtain and to cover her with the drape provided.

Then *position* the patient on the couch.

Ask her to keep her ankles together and gently drop her knees.

While the patient gets ready, have the slide prepared with the patient's name, hospital No. and DOB on the ground-glass end of the slide.

Put on the gloves.

Inspect the vulva and comment on its appearance (ulcer, discharge and skin redness).

Ensure that the speculum is warm and in good working order (if it was cold, warm by hot water).

Before touching the patient, ask her if she feels any pain?

Inform the patient that you are about to insert the speculum, it may be a bit uncomfortable.

Part the labia with the non-dominant hand (with 2 fingers) and insert the speculum with the blades closed and its lateral side parallel to vulva and when you are turning for 90°,

Again slightly withdraw it until the cervix comes to view.

Tighten the screw to secure its position.

Insert the smear spatula and rotate it through 360° over the cervix and make a second rotation.

Remove the spatula, spread the material onto the labelled glass slide using longitudinal strokes.

Immediately fixate it. Leave to be fixed for 10 minutes.

Loosen the screw, close the blades and gently remove the speculum form vagina.

Complete the request form with a ball pen.

Place the slide in a slide mailer for dispatch with the request form.

Thank the patient for her co-operation and inform her that the smear will be sent to a laboratory for examination and that she will be notified of the results by post.

If it was normal, she should then have routine cervical smear every 3 years until she is 60 years of age.

BLADDER CATHETERIZATION

Greet, introduce yourself and identify the patient.

Explain the procedure and its purpose.

"I'm going to introduce this tiny tube into your front passage to drain your water bag."

Obtain a verbal consent.

Ensure privacy and ask for chaperone.

Wash hands.

Check the equipments.

Catheter trolley contains:

- Foley's urethral catheter size 12.
- Antiseptic cleansing fluid.
- Sterile drapes.
- Sterile gloves (2 pairs).
- Forceps.
- Cotton balls.
- 10 ml syringe and 10 ml vial of normal saline.
- Lignocaine gel.
- Urine bag.

Prepare the syringe.

Put on a pair of gloves.

Sterilze

Hold the penis at right angle with the left hand.

Use forceps and cotton and antiseptic solution to sterile the penis:

1. Glance upper surface.
2. Glance lower surface.
3. Lower surface of the shaft of penis.
4. Upper surface of the shaft of penis.
5. Groin.

Drape with sterile paper towel drapes.

Instill Lignocaine gel inside the penis.

Apply gel to the tip of the catheter as well. (Wait for 5 minutes).

With the penis held at right angle, introduce the catheter gently and watch for urine.

Check the balloon volume and size and inflate it according to what is written.

Connect the exposed end of the Foley's catheter to the drainage bag.

Slowly retract the catheter until resistance is felt, when the inflated balloon comes to rest at bladder neck.

Tidy up yourself.

Explain that you would thank the patient for his co-operation.

Be fluent, confident and professional.

VENEPUNCTURE

Greet and introduce yourself.

Check the patient's identity on the bracelet.

Explain the procedure and its purpose.

Obtain a verbal consent.

Check your *equipment:*

- A pair of sterile gloves.
- Cotton.
- A vacutainer and its needle.
- Tourniquet.
- Alcohol steret.

Don the gloves.

Apply the tourniquet to the upper arm and proximal to the site of venepuncture not unnecessarily tight.

Ask the patient to make a fist, release it and to repeat the action.

(Consider gentle tapping if the vein was difficult to be seen.)

Select an appropriate vein by gentle palpation.

Cleanse the area with the alcohol street and wait until it dries.

Advise the patient to look away as you approach the cephalic or basilic or any other obvious veins.

Inform the patient that s/he will feel a sharp scratch.

Approach at an oblique 30°–45°,

Once the vein is pierced, reduce the angle to 15° and attach each tube to the inside of the vacutainer and the blood will be drawn directly into the tube by suction action.

Exchange the tube once full.

Release the tourniquet and cover the area with a piece of cotton gauze.

As you remove the needle, ask the patient to hold a pressure over the site for 3 minutes.

Safely dispose the needle to the sharp bin.

Ask the patient if he is allergic to Elastoplast; If not, place it; if yes, place a tape over the cotton.

Label the tubes as indicated with the patient's full name, hospital number DOB, your name, date, time and location.

Place the blood tubes in separate plastic bags and seal the bags.

Insert the appropriate blood form with each bag.

After recognizing that the patient is well, thank him/her for co-operation.

CANNULATION

Greet and introduce yourself.

Check the patient's identity on the bracelet.

Explain the procedure and its purpose.

Obtain verbal consent.

Check your equipment.

Intravenous cannula.

Alcohol wipe.

Tourniquet.

Vecafix.

10 ml syringe.

Normal saline flush.

Sterile gloves.

Don the gloves.

Apply the tourniquet to the upper arm.

Select a vein by gentle palpation of the antecubital fossa.

Cleanse the area with the alcohol steret and wait until it dries.

Palpate the vein with the fingers of your non-dominant hand and Slowly advance the cannula into the vein with your dominant hand at 35°–45°.

As soon as you see the blood return or the flash back.

Advance the plastic sheath while withdrawing the introducing needle.

Simultaneously, press on the tip of the cannula and ask the patient to raise the arm.

While your index finger on the plastic tube, remove the needle and put it in the sharp bin safely but remove the cap before putting the needle into the sharp bin.

Recap the venflon.

Secure the cannula with vecafix.

Fill the 10 ml syringe with normal saline from the 10 ml vial provided and flush the cannula slowly.

Thank the patient for his/her co-operation.

Be fluent, confident and professional.

SUTURING

Greet and introduce yourself.

Explain that the wound needs sutures.

Establish that there is full range of movement and there is no neurovascular compromise or tendon injury. Ask the patient to lie in supine position.

Check your requirements:

- A good source of light.
- Suturing materials.
- Lignocaine.
- Syringe.

Sterilize, each side in opposite direction (hold the cotton with the forceps).

Anaesthetize with 10 ml Lignocaine infiltration with 21 G needle 1–2 mm from the edge of the wound into under the dermis. Tell the patient that s/he may feel bee-sting sensation of the local anaesthetic. Withdraw suction of the needle before advancing the needle.

Wait until the area is fully anaesthetized (5–10 minutes).

Warn the patient that s/he will feel pressure but not pain.

Apply steristrips and sterile gauze dressing over the wound.

Inform the patient that the sutures will need to be removed in a week's time and that s/he should make arrangements at her local GP surgery to see the nurse for suture removal.

Inform the patient that if s/he develops signs of infection (temperature, wound breakdown, wound discharge), s/he should return to the casualty or to see her GP soon.

Give painkillers.

Consider immunization and vaccination against tetanus if indicated (if the patient was not immunised in the last 10 years or if the wound is contaminated).

Thank the patient for his/her co-operation.

Antiseptic solutions as hydrogen peroxide or Betadine.

Possible anaesthetic side effects:

1. Adrenaline can cause ischaemic tissue necrosis, so avoid its use in fingers, ear lobe and nose.
2. Massive intravenous dose of Lignocaine can cause convulsions, depression of CNS, heart block and acute heart failure.

CPR (BASIC LIFE SUPPORT) FOR ADULT

If you were alone, quickly check for the hazards for yourself "Am I safe?" and then for the hazards for the victim "Is the patient safe?".

Exclude the possibility of neck injury by asking the examiner "Any evidence of neck injury or cervical injury?"

Establish the patient is conscious by speaking to him/her loudly near his/her ears saying: "Are you alright? Are you alright? Are you alright?" and simultaneously by shaking his/her shoulders or tapping on his/her chest.

If there is no response, apply strong physical stimuli such as pinching his/her ears.

Shout loudly for help: "Help! Help! Help!".

Position the victim on his/her back on a hard surface.

Check the airways and clear them if there was any obstruction by a finger sweep.

Tilt head and lift chin.

Look, listen and feel for any breathing for 10 seconds " 1 and 2 and 3 and 4 and 5 and 6 and 7 and 8 and 9 and 10".

Activate the crash team. If you were outside the hospital mention that you'll dial 999 and ask for emergency resuscitation team and you'll give them the place address and you'll wave hands when they arrive. If you were inside the hospital, you simply activate the emergency resuscitation team activator button which is present in every ward.

Come back to the patient, pinch his/her nose and give 2 rescue breathes.

Check the carotid pulse for 10 seconds "1 and 2 and 3 and 4 and 5 and 6 and 7 and 8 and 9 and 10".

If there were no pulse and no breathing, start cardiac compressions: Identify the xiphoid process of the sternum, place the heel of your both hands 2 fingers above the process and give 15 compressions / 2 inflations at a rate 100 compressions / minute. The compression's power should be enough to compress the chest 4 cm downwards.

Check the carotid pulse every one minute from the first rescue breath.

If the patient moved or made a spontaneous breath, check for the carotid pulse for 10 seconds and give 5 rescue breaths if the patient stops from spontaneous breathing.

If the heart starts to beat but there was not breathing, continue inflations up to 5 breaths until spontaneous breathing resumes.

If the heart beating and breathing were resumed continuously, place the patient on recovery position, i.e. left lateral position.

Otherwise continue CPR until

The crash team arrives.

You are exhausted.

The victim recovers.

NB* If two people present, after the first 2 rescue breaths.

Compression / inflation ratio should be 5:1 without waiting after the inflations.

Never rely on pupil size before, during or after resuscitation.

You must not delay activation of crash team unless the victim is drowned, or injured, in which case you activate the team 1 minute after starting resuscitation.

CPR (BASIC LIFE SUPPORT) OF CHILD and INFANT

CPR of children > 8 years old is exactly the same as adult CPR.

In children 1–8 years old, the following differences should be recognised: Put hand over the forehead before shaking the child.

Activation of crash team should be delayed for 1 minute after starting inflations and compressions.

Compression / inflation ratio should be 5:1, after the first 2 rescue breaths.

For compressions, the heel of 1 hand should be used instead of 2 hands.

Compression force should be enough to compress the chest 2–3 cm downwards.

In infants i.e. 28 days to 1 year old, the following differences should be recognised: Put hand over the forehead of the infant before shaking.

Activation of crash team should be delayed for 1 minute after starting inflations and compressions.

Compression / inflation ratio should be 5:1, after the first 2 rescue breaths.

If there was spinal injury, do jaw thrust.

Seal your lips around both his/her mouth and nose to give inflations.

Check pulse at brachial artery.

Use two fingers for chest compressions.

Compression force should be enough to compress the chest 2 cm downwards.

BLOOD PRESSURE MEASUREMENT

Greet, introduce yourself and identify the patient.

Explain the procedure and its purpose. Has his BP been checked before? (Rest, no caffeine, no smoking).

While following the basic steps take a brief history of HTN, on any current medications which may cause postural hypotension.

Check the manometer set to zero.

Choose the correct sized cuff.

Check the inflation and deflation of the device.

Check service intervals / calibration.

Palpate the brachial artery to locate its site. Rap the cuff 2 cm above the antecubital fossa.

Inflate while palpating the radial artery until the pulse disappears (palpatory systolic blood pressure), inflate an extra 30 mmHg more, apply the diaphragm of the stethoscope on the brachial artery and deflate slowly 2 mm/second, record systolic and diastolic pressure accurately.

Take BP on standing as well (you do not need to measure palpatory again).

Thank the patient.

FUNDOSCOPY

Greet, introduce yourself and identify the patient.

Explain the procedure and its purpose: "I'm going to flash bright light into your eyes to have a look at the back of your eyes and during the examination I will come very near to your face."

Obtain verbal consent.

Ask for a chaperone.

Check the ophthalmoscope

Set the lens on not.

If the patient is hypermetropic, convex + lenses.

If the patient is myopic, concave - lenses.

Remove your spectacles, if you wear any.

Darken the room to dilate the pupils.

Ask the patient to look at straight ahead, use right hand to examine the right eye while lifting the lid with left hand fingers.

Look at front of the eye; look at the lens and vitreous and see.

Set on not. One foot away from the eye to see red reflex and lens opacity.

Then slowly move towards the patient to see any opacity in vitreous.

Look at the fundus

1. To the disc while the patient is looking straight ahead

   Contour of the disc (sharp or blurred).

Colour of the disc (pale or normal (pink)).

Cup size compared to the total size of the disc.

2. Around the disc: Pigmentery changes.

   Scleral crescent.

   Scleral rings.

3. Four quadrants of the retina (ask the patient to move his/her eye up and to the right), look for the vessel's (arteries and veins) calibre, crossing and the space in between them (haemorrhages, hard exudates, soft exudates and other abnormalities).

4. Macula (ask the patient to look directly at the light) the pupil should be dilated. Fovea {yellow foveal reflex (mainly in youngs), temporal to macula}. The area in which the earliest changes of diabetic maculopathy occurs.

Check the left eye.

Comment on your findings.

Thank the patient for his/her co-operation.

NB: Consider dilating the pupil to examine the macula (if it was difficult to be seen). Make sure that the patient is not driving himself home and that he has a companion to do so. Do not give long-acting mydriatics such as atropine, which has been known to last up to 21 days! It is illegal to drive with a dilated pupil. Use 0.5–1% Tropicamide, a short-acting mydriatic, that lasts for 3 hours.

Do not dilate the pupil of a patient with suspected angle closure glaucoma. In other words, beware of the elderly female who is long-sighted for she is more at risk of developing angle closure glaucoma.

BREAST EXAMINATION

First of all, you will greet the patient and introduce yourself. Then, you will explain the examination and ask for her permission. You will ensure her privacy and ask for a chaperone.

Tell the examiner that in real life and in any circumstances you shall examine and compare both the breasts.

Ask the patient to undress to waist and to sit on a chair.

Sit in front of her and start examination with inspection while:

- Her hands are resting on her thighs.
- She is pressing firmly on her hips.
- Her arms above her head.
- And finally, while she is leaning slightly forward, for any:
  - Asymmetry or local swelling,
  - Dimpling,
  - Peau d'orange,
  - Skin changes or lesions,
  - Nipple retraction or discharge.

(After this introduction to the examiner, start examination on the dummy.)

Examine one breast after the other and in each side do not forget:

- The breast tail,
- The nipple,

The areola.

Squeeze the nipples for any discharge.

Palpate for the texture of the breast and for any nodule, lump or mass. If any is present, describe it as follows:

Site (in which quadrant of which breast?)

Size (about .... × .... cm)

Consistency (soft, firm or stony hard)

Surface (smooth, regular or irregular)

Tender or not.

Mobile or fixed; attachment to the surrounding structures, i.e., overlying skin or underlying chest wall.

Palpate the axillary, the cervical and the supraclavicular lymph nodes in each side. Describe any palpable lymph node as follows:

Site

Size (about .... × .... cm).

Consistency (soft, firm or hard).

Tender or not.

Matted together or not.

Fixed to the surrounding structures or not.

Auscultate the chest.

Examine the abdomen for hepatomegally and ascites.

Percuss the spine.

Then tell the examiner that you want to end the examination by thanking the patient for her co-operation.

EAR EXAMINATION (OTOSCOPY)

First of all, I will greet the patient, introduce myself, explain the examination and ask for permission.

I shall make sure that the instrument is working well and I will choose the right 'speculum'.

Before I start, I have to examine the external ear and the lymph nodes of the head and neck.

I will start my examination by gently pulling the pinna upwards and backwards and inserting the speculum.

After looking at the external canal, I shall look at the eardrum and what I can see behind it (if there is a wax obstructing my vision, I have to remove it by wax hook or by gentle syringing with warm water).

Finally, I shall summarise my findings and give a differential diagnosis.

Common abnormalities in the examination.

The normal.

The tympanic membrane is thin and semi-transparent.

The handle of the malleus can be seen.

A cone of light extends downwards and forwards.

Wax or cerumen.

With time changes from pale yellow to golden yellow, to light brown and finally, black.

Can obscure or partially obscure the drum.

Acute otitis media with or without effusion.

Congested ear drum (prominent blood vessels).

Bulging of the ear drum.

Effusion (fluid levels, purulent fluid).

Perforation.

Serous (secretory) otitis media (glue ear).

The eardrum has lost its lustre.

Effusion is visible through the eardrum (fluid level).

The handle of the malleus is also difficult to visualise.

Resolution of middle ear effusion.

Tympanosclerosis.

In some cases of otitis media, healing may not be completed and the inflammatory process leads to the formation of scar tissue. This can take the form of calcified plaques on the tympanic membrane.

Central perforation of the ear drum.

Perforations are usually single but may be multiple.

Grommet (tympanostomy tube):

If medical treatment and myringotomy are unsuccessful and there is persistent middle ear effusion, a silicone tube is inserted and retained in the drum.

PHONE CONVERSATION

INTESTINAL OBSTRUCTION, CALL THE REGISTRAR

"Hello, Dr (Registrar), I am Dr (you), senior house officer in A and E.

I have a patient who is 72-year old female, she is presented with a history of abdominal pain of 24 hours duration.

The pain is central, was first colicky in nature then became more diffuse aching, she vomited twice, and has constipation since yesterday.

On examination (O/E)

She is conscious.

Pulse rate, blood pressure and temperature are normal" (mention figures according to those given in the exam chart).

Talk about signs of dehydration (according to instructions). Fluid input/output values. Abdomen is distended with tenderness all over the abdomen.

Investigations

"We took blood for FBC, U and E, blood chemistry. Results showed increased urea level, increased haematocrit, and increased globulin.

We did plain AXR, erect which showed multiple fluid level, the supine film showed dilated large bowel (ascending and transverse colon are located at the periphery. The haustra are on two-thirds the way from one wall to another and irregularly spaced."

N.B.: For small intestines valvulae conniventes were seen all the way from one wall to another, regularly spaced and located centrally. Barium enema and meal are contraindicated.

Management

1. "We put N/G tube to decompress the bowel and to prevent aspiration.
2. We give N/S to correct fluid and electrolyte imbalance.
3. We took blood for grouping and cross-match and save.
4. We gave antibiotic cefuroxime.
5. Analgesia, morphine."
6. "Why do you call me?" "Because I suspect intestinal obstruction with strangulation (may be right inguinal hernia), and an urgent surgery may be indicated."

RIGHT HEMICOLECTOMY, CALL YOUR REGISTRAR

"Hello, this is Dr ...., the surgical SHO on duty.

I am on ward 14 and I have been called to see a patient of Mr (consultant).

The patient's name is Mr/Mrs/Ms (patient), he/she is 59 year old, who had a right hemicolectomy procedure done 6 hours ago by Mr (consultant), due to localised neoplasm of the bowel.

From the operation note it seems that the operation was relatively straight-forward and that there was no macroscopic evidence of metastasis outside the colon. The liver, lymph nodes seemed clean and there was no ascites.

She came from recovery about an hour after the operation. The results of her monitoring were fine until about an hour ago. Over the last hour her blood pressure dropped from 120/80 mmHg, to 90/60 mmHg/min.

I am not sure of what is going on, but it looks most likely that she is bleeding and may have to be taken back to the theatre."

Action taken

"I asked the nurses to continue the quarter-hourly observation.

The laboratory already has serum grouped and saved. I have asked them to cross match four units of blood and Haemaccel.

I have already started oxygen by mask and infusion.

She is already on heparin and has no chest pain, cough nor problems with her leg to suggest DVT and PE.

She has a history of mild angina and I am arranging to do ECG.

She is already on cephaloridine and metronidazole.

I tried to get in touch with Mr (consultant) but he has not answered my bleep.

I think you need to see her within ½ hour or so, I have feeling that she has bleeding and we may need to take her back to the theatre. And I have not done anything about it yet.

Are you going to be late. If so, would you like me to contact the theatre and anaesthetist on duty or would you like to see her first?

Right hemicolectomy is not doing well. Her blood pressure decreased and pulse rate increased. What would you tell her on telephone, on ward and after examining the patient.

I am now examining a patient in the casualty, but I will come as soon as I can." (You go to the ward as soon as possible.)

"Who was the nurse who bleeped me about the patient whom she was worried about?"

"The one who is now six hours after having right hemicolectomy and now he/she is unwell?"

"The nurse said that that the patient's name was Mrs Simpson. In which bed is she?" (make sure that you see the right patient).

Check the case sheet for the notes (history and examination) and read the operation note.

Then go to bed, check the chart, take brief history and any exam needed. (Check the abdomen, and auscultate heart, lung, and look at the legs.)

"I think she may be bleeding and she may have to go back to theatre.

1. I am just arranging for some blood to be cross-matched for her.
2. I will be getting in touch with the registrar on duty.
3. Could you change the drip to Haemaccel. I will write this in the chart. She is already on antibiotics and heparin, so I don't think that we need to give her anything else at present.
4. Could you make sure that the observations are taken regularly every 15 minutes?
5. Can you please tell me where I can find the ECG machine? I have not contacted the theatre or anaesthetist yet. I thought I would better to wait until she has been seen by the registrar, but it seems pretty likely that she may need to go back to the theatre.
6. Do you know if any of her relatives are here? I need to speak to them."

"Good morning, I am Dr (you), the doctor on duty.

As far as I know you are Mrs Simpson's daughter.

I need to have a word with you." (Take her to a side room).

"What is your name?

So Ms .... (the daughter), your mother's operation went very well and we think that we have removed all of her growth.

However, unfortunately, she developped another problem, which we think will only be temporary. It seems possible that she may be bleeding.

We arranged for her to have blood transfuson and hopefully that will be enough. But we may need to take her back to theatre.

You know this may happen sometimes, but should not make any difference in the long-term. She should be well. As soon as we know more, I will let you know. I am sorry but I have to go to sort things out."

POST-OPERATIVE COLLAPSE

Introduction

"Hello, this is Dr ...., the SHO on duty.

I am calling to tell you that I've been called to see Mr ...., age........., who had right hemicolectomy. He was fine until .... when his BP dropped from......mmHg to......mmHg."

ABC—Assess **A**irway, **B**reathing and **C**irculation.

With the aid of the nurse, administer 100 % oxygen by facemask.

Raise the foot end of the bed.

Insert 2 wide bore IV cannula.

Simultaneously take blood for typing.

Cross match 2 units of blood.

FBC.

Clotting,

UandE and glucose.

ECG / Urgent portable chest and abdominal X-ray.

Give Hartmann's solution fast.

Insert Foley's catheter.

Input and Output chart.

Ensure that a nurse will recheck the vital signs.

History, operative note, vital signs chart and drug chart.

Examine from the head to toe.

Pupil asymmetry, response to light and accommodation.

Auscultate the chest for pneumonia and heart failure.

Abdomen: peritoneal signs bleeding (tense abdomen, no bowel sound).

Do PR for bleeding.

Please come urgently to review the patient.

Prepare her for theatre and obtain verbal consent from her next of kin.

Inform theatre and the anaesthetist on call.

Transfuse two units of blood ASAP and type and cross match further four units of blood.

CHILD WITH DIARRHOEA

"Hello, this is Dr ....

How can I help you?

How old is he?

How long has he been like this?

How many times does he open his bowel?

Is it watery, loose or semi-formed?

Any blood, mucus, pus? (*mucus* = slippery) or pus?

Any tummy pain or lump?

Has he been sick?

How is he feeding?

Any fever?

Have you added any new type of food to his diet?

Has he been sick?

Any recent travel to abroad?"

Ask about sings of dehydration

"How is his mouth?

His tongue, is it dry or moist?

Or cry without tears?

His eyes seem to be depressed (sunken)?

Does he pass water as usual, frequency (weight of napies in infants)?

How is his breathing?"

In an infant, ask for depressed soft spot on scalp (anterior fontanelle)?

Then if the dehydration is mild, give him oral rehydration solution (ORS)

If ORS is not available, teach the mother how to prepare one:

1 L of water (2 pints of water), boil and let to cool, then add 10 teaspoons (TSF) of sugar and 1 TSF of salt.

And give the child by spoons as much as he accepts.

Don't give ORS if breastfeeding continues.

"Is everything clear? Any questions?"

HISTORY TAKING

IDDM - ANNUAL CHECK UP

Measure body weight.

Examine the *eyes* for:

Xanthelasma and arcus

Visual acuity (maculopathy)

Eye movements (mononeuritis multiplex, III, IV, VI cranial nerves)

Cataract

Rubeosis iridis

Ophthalmoscopy (retinopathy, vitrous haemorrhage)

Examine the *mouth* for candidiasis.

Neck

Listen for carotid bruit (atherosclerosis).

Upper limb examination

Blood pressure sitting and standing for postural hypotension, hypertension.

Radial pulse for resting tachycardia.

Inspect hands for wasting of thenar (carpal tunnel syndrome), hypothenar and interossei muscles (ulnar nerve palsy), inspect prick sites for infection, and ask the patient to do prayer sign (joint contracture).

Chest

Auscultate for signs of pneumonia, tuberculosis (TB) or congestive cardiac failure (CCF).

Lower limb examination

Please, see 'Essential Physical Examination' material, page 25.

NB: In DM early sensory loss includes vibration, deep pain and temperature while late sensory loss is joint position sensation (proprioception).

Investigations

Glycosylated Hb **(Hb A1c)** relates to blood glucose level over 6–8 weeks (normal: 2.3–6.5%).

Glycosylated plasma proteins (fructosamine) relates to blood glucose level over 1–3 weeks.

Urine analysis for: glucose, ketones and albumin (macro- and micro-albuminuria)

Blood for plasma creatinine and lipids.

Questions to ask

Ask about symptoms of hypoglycaemia.

Talk about general and specific problems.

Review of self-monitoring results and injection techniques.

Review of eating habit.

Education (nature of the disease and better ways of copying with it).

CHEST PAIN

Introduction.

"As far as I know, you have pain in your chest.

I would like to ask you several questions concerning your complaint.

It will take only a few minutes."

DPSRNAR

1. How long has the pain been there? (duration)
2. Is it there all the time or does it come and go? (periodicity)
3. Can you tell me exactly where it is? (site)
4. Does it spread? (radiation)
5. Can you describe it, what it feels like? (nature)
6. Does anything seem to make it worse? (Aggravating factors like: walking in cold weather, heavy meal, climbing stairs or hill)
7. How much can you do before you have to stop? Do you ever feel pain or discomfort at rest?
8. Does anything seem to make it better? (relieving factors)
9. Any shortness of breath, cough, sputum and fever? (pneumonia)
10. History of traveling abroad or prolonged sitting? (pulmonary embolism)
11. History of increase in pain after taking food or being hungry for long time? (peptic problem)

12. Positive family history, smoking history, obesity. (MI)
13. Any history of trauma or fall (muskuloskeletal pain).

Past history

Any history of similar complain.

History of hypertension, asthma.

Family history.

Similar complains in family.

Examination

1. Check vital signs: Temperature, pulse rate, respiratory rate, and blood pressure.
2. Auscultate the heart and lung bases.
3. Ask the patient to take a deep breath and cough (pain aggravates in patient with pleurisy).

Auscultate the area of pain and do vocal resonance.

Thank the examiner and the patient.

State the entire positive finding at the end of history and say that you suspect ....

If the station requires you to discuss the diagnosis with the patient or the examiner: "I would like to ask more question, do full examination and do needful investigation but due to lack of time, on the basis of my history I suspect the patient has ...."

D/D

1. MI
2. Pulmonary embolism
3. Pleuritic pain
4. Gastric/duodenal ulcer
5. Reflux oesophagitis
6. Trauma

PALPITATION

Introduction.

"How can I help you? I understand that you feel that your heart is racing;

I need to ask you a few questions about that. Is that alright?"

1. Onset
2. Duration
3. Progression
4. Aggravation factor
5. Relieving factor

"Where and when does it come on? (After exercise or at rest?)

What do you mean by palpitation?

Can you describe it for me, please?

Is it fast or slow?

Regular or irregular?

Can you tap it on table for me, please?

Where and when do you usually feel it?

How long does it last?"

Anxiety

1. "Are you anxious about anything?
2. Any pins and needles feeling in your hands?
3. Do you have any stress at home or at work?
4. Any exams coming up? result?
5. Sweaty palms hyperventillation?"

Hyperthyroidism

Did you notice any change in your weight?

How is your appetite?

How is your bowel motion?

How is your period? Is it heavy?

Do you prefer hot or cold weather?

Any tremor?

Sweating more than usual?

Do you get easily irritabile?

Tiredness, any anaemia?

Past-medical history

- IHD? • Angina? • High blood fat? • Hypertension?
- DM? • Stroke? • Rheumatic fever?

On any medication?

(Salbutamol, β-blocker, digoxin, theophylline, caffeine)

Any known drug allergies?

Social history

Drinking coffee heavily?

Stress at home or at work?

Drinking alcohol?

Smoking?

Any recreational drugs? (Speed and Ecstasy)

Family history

(IHD, HT, DM, stroke, high blood fat.)

"Any questions?"

"Thank you very much for your co-operation."

DD

Arrythmias (AF, ventricular ectopics, SVTs).

Anxiety.

Mitral valve prolapse syndrome

Thyrotoxicosis.

Excessive coffee or tea drinking.

Phaechromocytoma.

Anaemia.

Panic attacks

Hypoglycaemic

History of diabetes

CVA/TIA

Greet

Introduce

Identify yourself.

Acknowledge and ask for verbal consent.

"I understand that you had a sensation of pins and needles in your hand.

I need to ask you a few questions about that,

Then I'll explain what to do next, is that alright?

Could you tell me what happened please?

When did that happen?

How long did it last?

Have you had any similar conditions in the past?

Have you had any weakness in the arm or leg?

What did make it worse?

What did make it better?

Any change or loss of vision? Any double vision?

(VISION GOES OFF AS FALLING CURTAIN)

Any giddiness or dizziness?

Any difficulty with hearing?

Any ringing in your ears?

Any difficulty with speaking?

Do you have any headache?

Have you had any loss of consciousness? Blackouts?

Any trauma to your head?

Do you have any pain in your neck?

Any pain in your joints or heart problem?

Felt sick? Been sick?

Any difficulty with swallowing and chewing?

Any muscle shaking? Wasting? Twitching?

Any problem with walking?"

Past-medical

"Hypertension?

DM?

Heart problems?

High blood fat?

Stroke?

DVT?

PE?

Clotting abnormality?"

On any medication?

"Do you use OCP?

Are you on HRT?

Anticoagulant?"

Family history

"Has anyone else in your family had similar conditions?

Hypertension?

DM?

Heart problems?

High blood fat?
Stroke?"

Social history
"Drinking alcohol?
Smoking?"

Diet
"Do you have a lot of fatty meals or salt?
Any stress at home or at work?
Any questions?"
"Thank you very much for your co-operation."

PANIC ATTACK / HISTORY

Greet, introduce, identify, acknowledge and ask for consent.

"I understand that you are worried too much about things. Would you mind talking about that?

Could you tell me what do you think?

Where you usually get worried?

How do you feel then?"

GIT

Dry mouth.

Feeling of a lump in throat and chocking (difficulty in swallowing).

Epigasatric disturbance.

Butterflies in stomach, funny feeling in tummy.

Loose motions.

CVS

Chest pain.

Heart is racing? (awareness of the heart beat)

Sweating.

CNS

Tingling sensation (pins and needles).

Trembling of the hands.

Giddiness.

Feeling of impending doom.

Fear to sleep.

Respiratory

Tightness in chest

Difficulty in breathing

Over-breathing

"What makes you feel better?

What makes you feel worse?

How long have you been like this?"

Marriage and Socio-economic status

"Do you have a partner?

Any problems with him/her?

Are you worried about your children?

What do you do for living?

Have you got any problems or stress at home or at work?

Do you have any problems in getting to sleep and to relax?"

Psychiatric

"How do you feel in yourself?

Do you feel low?

Do you feel life is worth living?

Do you sleep late at night?

Wake up early at morning?

How is your appetite?

Felt sick? Been sick?

Have you lost weight?

Did you have any thoughts to harm yourself?

Have you planned for that? Attempted for that?

Did you left any notice? What did you write down?

Do feel sorry about that or you still want to try in future?

Do you find yourself to do things repeatedly? for example, washing hands.

Have you experienced unusual perceptions? (hallucinations)

Did you notice any thoughts controlling your mind? (delusions)"

Past-medical and past-psychiatric history

"Do you drink alcohol? (alcohol withdrawal)

Any recent dislikes of hot weather? (thyrotoxicosis)

Any high blood pressure? (phaeochromocytoma)

DM? (hypoglycaemia)

MVP?

If female: Any change in your periods?"

Medication history

"On any medication?

Valium withdrawal?

Recreational drugs?"

Family history

"Any mental illness in your family?"

Social

"Someone passed away?

Moving house?

Smoking?

Drinking coffee heavily?"

Management

Reassure the patient.

Relaxation training.

Psychotherapy (cognitive and behavioural therapy).

Medications: Benzodiazepines as Diazepam.

"Any questions?"

RECTAL BLEEDING

Introduction.

"I understand that you are passing blood from your back passage.

I need to ask you few questions then we will talk about what we will do next.

Could you tell me how old are you?

How long have you had that bleeding? (acute or chronic).

How much blood did you pass?

Is the blood mixed or on the surface of the stool?

Can you tell me the colour of the blood; is it bright red, dark red or black?

Does the blood come before, during or after passing motion?

Do you feel urge to pass motion?

Do you feel the need to pass motion and when you try nothing comes out?

Any blood on the toilet paper or pants?

Do you have any pain during passing motion?

Have you passed any pus, mucous or discharge with stool?

Did you notice any lump passing from your back passage? Prolapse, if yes, how does it go inside?

Associations: Tummy pain?

Any change in bowel habit? (colorectal carcinoma) Any diarrhoea?

Fainting attack? (severe bleeding)7

Constipation?

Joint pain, eye discharge-IBD

Distension of your tummy?

Passing wind more than usual?

Itching in the perianal region? (haemorroids)

Pain in the perianal region? (fissure)

Felt sick? Been sick?

How is your appetite?

Any weight loss?

Do you have bleeding from other site?

Past-medical history

"Have you had similar conditions in the past

Are you on any medication?" (anticoagulants)

Family history

"Has anyone in your family had similar condition?

Any bowel disease or tumour in your relatives? (bowel polyps)"

Social History

Diet:

"Do you eat a lot of vegetables and fruits?

Drinking alcohol?

Smoking?

Recent travel to abroad?

Sexual preferences: proctitis in gays?"

Investigations

FBC and coagulation profile

Stool examination

PR

Sigmoidoscopy

Any masses in the abdomen

D/D

Colorectal cancer

Haemorroids

Fissure in ano

Diverticulosis

Ulcerative colitis

General bleeding disorder

Rectal polyp

Trauma

SUICIDE / HISTORY

Introduce.

"I understand that you have tried to harm yourself.

You must be going through a difficult time.

Would you mind telling me why is that?

1. How did you plan for that?
2. Where?
3. When?
4. What did you use to harm yourself?

   (If tablets, ask about name, number of tablets, how many types of tablets.)
5. How long have you been planning this?
6. Did you leave a note? What did you write down?
7. How do you feel about what you did?
8. Have you ever tried to harm yourself before that?
9. If you've been discharged, what are you going to do?"

Personal background

What sort of person you were?.

Past-psychiatric and past-medical history?

On any medication?

Family background

1. Have you enjoyed your childhood?
2. Were you brought up by your parents?

3. Family bonding: Did you love your family members?
4. Is there any history of psychiatric illness in your family?
5. Any histories of deliberate self-harming in your family?"

Social history

"Any problem with your job or financial constraints?

Drinking alcohol?

Smoking cigarette?

Recreational drugs?

Speed (metamphetamine) or cannabis?"

DYSPHAGIA

Greet, introduce, identify the patient, acknowledge and ask for consent.

I understand that you have difficulty in swallowing,

I need to ask you few questions about that.

To see what is wrong, is that alright?

Could you please tell me more about that?

When you first noticed that?

Was it for food first (oesophageal), or for fluids (pharyngeal), or for both (achalasia or neurological causes) from the beginning?

Is it intermittent (oesophageal spasm) or it's constant and getting worse (malignant stricture)?

Do you have pain on swallowing? (cancer, oesophagitis, achalasia or oesophageal spasm).

Is there any bulging or gurgling in your neck on swallowing? (pharygeal pouch)

Do you cough on swallowing? (bulbar palsy)

At what level does the food appear to stick?

Do you repeat the food?

Or does the food eventually pass down?

Do you have pain in your chest?

Do you have any heartburn on lying down at night?

Have you got any temperature?

Any cough or chest pain?

Any chest infections in the past?

Any tummy pain?

Felt sick? Been sick? Did it contain blood?

Any change in the colour of your motions?

Any change in voice? (pharyngeal Ca, bulbar palsy

Is it difficult to co-ordinate the swallowing movement? (bulbar palsy)

Do you have any weakness in your face?

Do you get muscle weakness on repeating actions? (myasthenia gravis)

How is your appetite?

Do you have any weight loss? (oesophageal Ca)

Do you feel getting tired easily?

Night sweats?

Any skin changes and/or joint pain? (systemic sclerosis).

Any similar conditions in past?

Past-medical history (lung Ca, goitre, aortic aneurysm, left atrial enlargement)?

Past-surgical history? Radiotherapy? Corrosives?

Any family history of similar conditions? Anyone in your family has any other illness? (Ca)

On any medications?

Social history

Smoking?

Drinking alcohol?

Any recreational drugs? Work?

Any questions?"

"Thank you very much for your co-operation."

Investigations

1. FBC (anaemia).
2. U and E (dehydration).
3. CXR (mediastinal fluid level, absent gastric bubble, aspiration).
4. Barium swallow.
5. Upper GI endoscopy and biopsy.
6. Oesophageal manometry (if normal barium swallow).

ENT opinion, if suspected pharyngeal cause.

20 YRS FEMALE, RIGHT ILIAC FOSSA PAIN

Greet, introduce, identify, acknowledge and ask for consent.

"Could you describe the pain for me please?

It started suddenly or gradually?

Could you tell me where exactly the pain is?

How long it has been there? How severe it is?

Have you had any similar condition in the past?

How does it feel like?

Is it intermittent or is it constant and getting worse?

Is it there all the time or does it come and goes?

Does it go anywhere?

Is it tender?

Anything make it worse? (movement)

Anything make it better? (lying down or rolling around)

Medication?"

Associations

"Any bleeding from your down below? (colour, amount, consistency, bleeding from other sites, feeling dizzy)

Was it before or after the pain?

Periods? Partner? Contraception?

Any discharge from your down below?

Any possibility to be pregnant?
Any pain during intercourse?
How is your appetite?
What kind of diet you eat?
Feeling sick? (nausea).
Being sick? (vomiting).
Any change in the bowel habit?
Any change in the colour of the motions? (blood)
Any recent temperature?
Passing water more than usual?
Any burning sensation while passing water?
Any change in the colour of urine?
Any lump in your tummy?"

Past-Obstetric history?
"Been pregnant before?
Any miscarriages or termination of pregnancy?
Any history of pregnancy outside the womb?
Any problems during or after the delivery?
Past-medical history?
Past-surgical history?
On any medications? (warfarin, asprin).
Family history of similar conditions?
Social history – Smoking? Alcohol? Stress? Occupation?"

"Any questions?
Thank you very much for your co-operation."

D/D

Ectopic pregnancy.

Torted ovarian cyst.

Acute appendicitis.

Abortion.

BABY BLUES, POST-NATAL DEPRESSION

Introduce yourself and ask for consent.

"I understand that you are finding life a bit difficult, could you tell me what has been going on?

Onset?

Does the patient have insight to her complaint?

How do you feel in yourself? Do you feel low?"

Symptoms of depression

"Do you feel tired?

How is your sleep?

Do you cry often?

Do you enjoy things you used to enjoy before?

How is your appetite?"

Special questions

"Do you have any concerns about your health or your baby's health?

Do you think you or someone else may harm the baby?

Do you think life is worth living nowadays?

Have you been thinking about harming yourself? Or planned for that? Or attempted to do that?"

Risk factors

"Age?

Premorbid personality?

Childhood?

Have you felt like this in your previous pregnancies?

Have you had any problems in your previous pregnancies? (Stillbirth or miscarriages.)

History of the current pregnancy : Any problems?

How do you feel about your baby?

Have you being breastfeeding your baby in the last 3 months?"

Past-psychiatric history

"Is anyone in your family suffering from a psychiatric illness or mood problems?

Have you been feeling low before?

Do you suffer from PMT?"

Social History

"Partner?

Relation with the partner?

Do you feel any support from your family and friends?

Feeling isolated?

Are you working? Having stress with your job?"

AMENORRHOEA OF 9 MONTHS

Greet, introduce yourself and identify the patient.

Acknowledge.

"How old are you?"

Periods

1. "How old were you when you had your first period?
2. Were they regular from then?
3. If she was old, concentrate on asking the post-menopausal symptoms."

"Partner?

Contraception?

Pregnancy? any possibilities of being pregnant?

Past-Obstetric history

1. Past pregnancy? "Have you become pregnant before?"
2. Ever had any miscarriages before?
3. TOP?
4. D and C?
5. If she gave birth before.
   - I - Deliveries were normal?
   - II - Bleeding following deliveries? (Sheehan's syndrome)

Tired? Sleepy? Having temperature recently? (general illness)

Weight change? On any special kind of diet? Appetite? (anorexia nervosa and illness).

Depression

"How have you been feeling in yourself for the last year?"

Weight loss, mood changes, late sleeping and early wakening.

Identify the cause of the depression.

Endocrine

Hyperthyroidism

1. Dislike of hot weather?
2. Sweating?
3. Shaking (tremor)?
4. Frequent loose motions?

POS

1. Recent hair growth on the face, breasts and tummy?
2. Deepening of the voice? (virilization)
3. Weight gain?

Hyperprolactinaemia

1. Milky discharge from the nipples?
2. Disturbance of vision?

On any medications?

Past-medical History

Any history of chronic illness?

Any pain or mass in the tummy?

Social history

Any stress at home or at work?

Having a good relationship with family and friends?

Any change in environment (moving house)?

Any breavement?

EMERGENCY CONTRACEPTION

Greet, introduce, identify, acknowledge and ask for consent.

"I understand that you are worried because you think you will be pregnant.

I need to ask you few special and personal questions and we will talk about what to do next, whatever you say to me will be strictly confidential.

Is that alright?"

Reassure the patient, maintain a good eye contact and listen attentively.

Why do you think you are pregnant?

When did you last have sex?

Did he penetrate you?

Did you use condoms? Did the condom burst?

Have you got a partner? Is he well? (No STD?)

When did you start menstruating?

Were your periods regular?

How long do they last?

Are they heavy?

When the first day of your last period?

Any unprotected sex since then?

Are you on any type of contraception?

If yes, why do you think it has failed?

Did you take emergency contraception before?

Have you ever had been treated for STDs?

Have you ever been pregnant before?

Any medical illnesses as blood clotting disorders?

Migraine? PID?

On any medications? (anti-epileptics or antibiotics)"

Social history

Smoking?

Drinking alcohol?

Discuss the methods of emergency contraception by using

Levonelle-2 -SEs are feeling sick and being sick, cause some delay in your next period 10%

OR

Coil (IUCD)-SEs tend to be expelled in those women who have never given birth, pregnancy outside the womb, PID and infertility, cause heavy painful periods.

Contraindicated in HIV,

Wilsons and heart disease.

Discuss the small risks of failure.

Levonelle: 95% active in < 24 hours.

85% between 24 and 48 hours.

58% between 48 and 72 hours.

Coil: 99% active within 1st–5th day.

Discuss the need for long-term contraception until her next period.

Have a non-judgemental and open attitude.

Any other concerns?

"Thank you very much for your co-operation."

VAGINAL BLEEDING

Introduce yourself.

"You didn't have your periods for the last 8 weeks, and now you have bleeding from your down below.

I would like to ask you some questions, and then I will explain to you what we will do."

You may ask her if it is OK, then proceed with your questions.

"When did the bleeding happen?

Can you describe the bleeding for me?

Is it bright red? (abortion).

Or dark red or brown? (ectopic pregnancy).

Is it heavy bleeding with clots or just slight blood loss?

Have you felt any pain in your tummy? (site, and character).

Have you always had regular periods?

Do you think you might be pregnant?

Do you feel sick?

Is there any pain in your breasts?

Did you notice if your breasts enlarged lately?

Do you use any contraceptive method?

What kind you use? IUCD, pills? (IUCD, progesteron only pill risk ectopic pregnancy)

Have you ever had ectopic pregnancy?

Have you ever had previous miscarriages?

Have you ever had vaginal discharge?

Any recurrent pain in the lower part of your tummy? (PID)

Have you ever had any previous operation in your tummy? (appendectomy,C/S)

How have you been feeling in yourself recently?

Any stress in job or at home?

Have you experienced any pain between shoulder blades?

Do you have any pain when passing water?

Any burning sensation?

How is your bowel motion?

Do you have any medical problem?

Do take any medication?

Do you have any bleeding from other sites?

Have you suffered any dizziness? Have you fainted?

Now I would like to examine you, and after exam we need to run some tests, especially pregnancy test, to make sure if you are pregnant or not.

And we need to do ultrasound examination to be sure that the possible pregnancy is in the right place, which is in your womb.

Don't worry, you will be all right, we will look after you."

Associations

1. Weight loss?

2. Loss of appetite and energy?

ROS

1. Back pain?

2. Bowel motion changes?

Medications

1. Tamoxifen?
2. HRT?

Family history of breast Ca and endometrial Ca?

Social history (smoking and alcohol)?

YOUNG LADY, VAGINAL BLEEDING AND LEFT ILIAC FOSSA PAIN

Introduce yourself, and you may continue by saying: "As far as I know, you have bleeding from your down below, and you feel pain in the left lower part of your tummy. I would like to ask you a few questions about your condition."

"Can you describe the bleeding for me?

Is it bright red? (miscarriage)

Or dark red or brown? (ectopic pregnancy)

Is it heavy bleeding with clots?

How many tampons (or pad) you use?

Is it heavy bleeding (miscarriage), or slight blood loss? (ectopic pregnancy).

Can you tell exactly where the pain is?

Can you tell what it feels like?

Did the pain start before bleeding? (ectopic pregnancy).

Or you saw bleeding before feeling pain? (miscarriage).

How were your periods: Regular or irregular?

Have you ever had unprotected sexual contact?

Do you think you are pregnant?

Do you feel sick? Is there any breast discomfort, pain, or enlargement?

Do you use contraception? What kind? (IUCD and progesterone only pills in ectopic pregnancy)

Have you ever had ectopic pregnancy before?

Any miscarriages?

Have you ever had vaginal discharges before?

Or recurrent pain in lower part of your tummy?

Have you ever had any operation before, especially in your tummy?" (ask about appendectomies, Cesarean section)

D/D

1. Ectopic pregnancy
2. Miscarriage (threatened or inevitable).
3. Chronic PID.
4. Dysfunctional uterine bleeding.

SCAPHOID FRACTURE

Introduction.

"As far as I know you have pain in your right hand since yesterday." Ask for site, radiation, aggravating and relieving factors, any associated symptoms and severity.

Inspection

Any swelling, deformity or bruises on the radial side of wrist.

Palpation

Palpate for tenderness over the carpal bones in general, then in the anatomical snuff box, and apply axial pressure on the extended thumb or index finger.

Movement

Ask the patient to flex and extend the wrist.

Look for pain.

Investigation

Request X-ray: Anteroposterior, lateral, and 2 oblique views.

Diagnosis

Fracture of scaphoid bone.

Management

If the fracture appears on the X-ray, then immobilise in scaphoid plaster for around 8 weeks.

ıf no fracture appears on X-ray, and scaphoid fracture is strongly suggested on clinical ground then apply scaphoid plaster for 2 weeks.

Repeat X-rays

I fracture is detected, then use plaster for 8 weeks. If fracture doesn't appear and if bone scan is available, then you may use it.

Also, give the patient analgesic for pain relief.

Some surgeons prefer internal fixation.

Complications

Malunion.

Avascular necrosis.

Osteoarthritis.

GOUT

Introduction.

"As far as I know you have pain in your foot. I would like to ask you a few questions about your condition."

"How long has the pain been there? (duration)

Is it there all the time or does it come and go? (periodicity)

Can you tell me exactly where the pain is? (site)

Does it spread? (radiation)

Is it painful when you touch it, any swelling, any redness?

Do you feel any heat over the toe? (septic arthritis)

Do you have pain in other joints? Any skin rash? (SLE)

Any redness of eye or pain on passing water? (Reiter's syndrome).

Do you have any tummy pain? Have you had a similar pain before?"

For gout ask

"Did you have any accident, injury, or surgery?

Do you have any disease (blood disease, rheumatoid arthritis, osteoarthritis)?

Do you have any kind of problem? Passed stone before with water?

Are you on any medication? (aspirin, diuretics)

Are you on any diet? Do you eat a lot of red meat?

Do you drink at all? How much of alcohol?

Has anyone else in your family had similar condition? Any kind of problem?"

POST-TRAUMATIC DISORDER

Introduction.

"I have heard that you had an accident recently, and you feel low now. Could you tell me more about this accident?"

"When did it happen?

How did it happen?

Do you think it was just an accident?

Who were with you?

Was anyone injured in the accident?

What were you thinking at time of accident?

Could you tell me more about the morning of the accident?

Did you have any problem with your family?

Any stress? Were you feeling low then?

When did you start to feel low?

Before the accident or after?

Is it your first time?

Do you drink? How much?"

Symptoms of depression:

Loss of interest or pleasure,

loss of appetite,

loss of weight,

early wakening,

diurnal variation in mood,

loss of interest in sex,

psychomotor retardation (slowness),

loss of concentration,

worthlessness,

feeling of guilt,

suicidal thoughts.

"Do you think life is worth living?

Have you felt so low that you have considered harming yourself?

Have you had thoughts of harming yourself?

Do you like to be with people or do you prefer to be alone?

Do you smoke?

Do you drink?

Do you take any drugs?"

Present circumstances

"Do you have any problem at work or with money?

Do you have any problem with your partner or at home?

Did you have any recent bereavement?"

Past and family history

"Did you have any mental illness? Other illnesses?

Any mental or other illnesses in the family?

Do take any medication?

Birth, growth and development?

How were you at school?

Did you have many friends?

What are your hobbies? Sport? Reading?

Did you have any trouble with the Law?"

Pre-morbid personality

"How have you been feeling in yourself?

It is quite natural for people to feel low when they have an accident.

We can give you some help by referring you to one of my colleagues who is a specialist in this area."

PNEUMONIA

Introduction.

"What seems to be troubling you? (The patient complains of chest pain and fever)

How long have you been like this (feverish)?

Do you have fever all the time or does it come and go?

Do you have any chills or sweating?

Could you tell me more about your chest pain where it is exactly?

Does it spread anywhere?

Can you describe what it feels like?

What brings the pain on?

Does anything seem to make it better or worse?

Do you have cough?

Any phlegm? (amount, smell, and colour)

Any blood with phlegm?

Do you have shortness of breath?

Any wheeze or noisy breathing?"

Atypical pneumonia

"Do you have headache, joint pain and muscle pain?

Have you been sick?

Do you have frequent bowel motions?

Bleeding from any site?

Do you keep birds at home like parrots, pigeon or turkey?

Did you travel abroad recently?
Did you stay in a hotel?"

Questions for predisposing factors for pneumonia

Do you have any problem with your lung, asthma and frequent flues?

Do you have any diseases, DM, heart disease?

Have you been admitted to hospital recently?

Do you take any medication?

Do you have any allergy?

Do you smoke? How many cigarettes a day?

Do you take any IV drugs?

"Well, Mr .... you seem to have a chest infection which could be pneumonia, but first we need to run some tests. We are going to take a tiny drop of your blood and do CXR for you and I will see you again after that."

ASTHMA

Introduction.

"You have asthma, and you got shortness of breath many times in the last 3 months, charac by recurrent episode of dyspnoea, cough and wheeze."

"How long have you had asthma?

Do you use peak flow meter?

Were you admitted in emergency anytime?

How frequently you have been getting it?

Is your shortness of breath more likely to occur in the morning, afternoon or evening?

Does it affect your sleep?

Do you wake up short of breath?

Is it more likely to occur in weekdays or weekends?

Did you have sick leave from work because of shortness of breath?

Do you feel short of breath when you walk or climb stairs?

Did you have eczema, hay fever? (atopic disease)"

Assessing precipitating factors

(Check inhaler technique)

"What medication do you take for asthma?

Do you take your medication regularly?

Did you have any fever, cough, phlegm, flue and chest pain?

Do you take any other medications? B-agonists, NSAIDs?

Any stress at home or at work?

Under any emotional stress? (family, partner)

Did you change your work?

Acid reflux?

Any particular food precipitating it?

Seasonal variation? (more in winter)

Exercise?

Any drug allergy?

Did you change your accommodation?

Do you keep pets?

Do you have any new carpet, furniture, pillow or duvet?

Do you smoke and how many cigarettes?

Have you had any unusual exercise?"

Past History

Similar complain.

Personal History

Smoking.

Alchol.

Recreational drug.

HTN

DM

Family History

Asthama

Allergies

Trigger factors

Pollen, dust mould, pregnancy, menstruation, infection, stress, exercise, allergens, drugs, emotion, weather change, furry animals, dairy products, viral infection and cold air.

DIARRHOEA

Introduction.

"As far as I know you pass loose motion. I would like to ask you a few questions about your condition."

"How long have you had this?

How many times do you open your bowel?

Is it watery or loose stool?

Are these always watery or sometimes you get formed or hard stool?

Is there any blood, mucous, pus with the stool?

What colour is the blood? Is it bright red or dark?

Is it mixed with stool? (At the beginning of stool, at the end, or mixed with stool?)

Streaking of blood with stool? Quantity of blood?

Any unusual smell of the stool?

Fatty that is difficult to flush? (malabsorption)

Do you feel urge to pass motion?

Do you feel the need to open bowel and nothing comes?

Do you have any pain, while passing stool, in periumbilical region or in right iliac fossa?

Any wind?

Have you felt sick? Have you been sick? [acute watery diarrhoea, fever, nausea, vomitting, abdominal cramps, general malaise (infection)]

Have you lost weight recently? How is your appetite?

Change in bowel habit recently? any blood from back passage?

Diarrhoea alternating with constipation?

Incomplete bowel evacuation? (tenesmus, colorectal Ca)

Chronic or intermittent diarrhoea? (young women, stresed people)

Period of constipation interspersed with diarrhoea? (hard marble/pellet like stool, commonly in morning) Rectal urgency? (irritable bowel syndrome)

Do you have any fever?

Do you experience diarrhoea when fasting?

Do you have diarrhoea at night?

Which prescription or over the counter medications have you used recently? (antibiotics, bloodthinners — pseudomembranous colitis)

What are your social and sexual habits?

Have you traveled abroad recently? (amoebiasis)

Weight loss? Do you have any joint pain, skin rash, redness of eye? (IBD)

Has anyone else in your family had a similar condition? (food poisning)

Palpitation, sweating, amenorrhea, heat intolerance, appetite? (thyrotoxicosis)

Have you had similar condition in the past?"

Personal history

Smoking, alcohol, recreational drugs, HTN, DM.

Family history.

Similar complain, cancer of bowel.

Allergies, if any.

D/D

Inflammatory bowel disease as Crohn's disease and ulcerative colitis.

Infectious diseases as bacillary or amoebic dysentery.

Antibiotic membranous colitis

Hyperthyroidism

Traveller diarrhoea

Irritable bowel syndrome

Malabsorption

Colonic malignancy

Bowel resection

HIV infection

Diabetic neuropathy

Faecal impaction

Giardiasis

"To exclude others, I need to examine the abdomen and do PR and test for occult blood."

ANOREXIA

Introduction.

"I understand that you have some weight loss. I would like to ask you few questions about your condition."

"When did you notice that you were losing weight?

What was your weight before that?

And what is your weight now?

Over how long or through how much time you lost that amount of weight?"

Associations

"Do you have fever?

Energy and tiredness?

Sleep?

Cough?

SOB?

Chest pain?

Do you open your bowel frequently? (diarrhoea)

Do you notice that the waste couldn't be flushed away easily? (steatorrhea)

Do you feel thirsty? Passing water frequently? (DM)

Any recent intolerance of heat? Sweating and tremor? (hyperthyroidism)

How is your appetite?

Do you take any special diet?"

Psychiatric

"Do you think that you are thin?
Have usual weight or overweight?
Do you ever induce vomiting?
Use any medication to decrease weight?
Do you exercise to lose weight?
Do you feel low?
Do you think life is worth living?
How do you feel in yourself?
What about your periods? Are they regular?
Any mood changes during day?
Still enjoy things you used to like them before?"

Social

"Any job (ballet dancer) or home stress?
Drinking?
Smoking?
Past-medical and past-psychiatric history?
On any medication?
Do you take any medication to decrease weight?
Do you take any recreational drugs?"

Family history

"Any history of psychiatric illness in your family?"

HAEMATURIA

Greet, introduce yourself and identify the patient.

"I understand that you pass blood with water. I need to ask you few questions, then we will discuss what to do next, is that OK?".

"Could you tell me please what has been going on?

How long have you been passing blood with water? (frank, passing of clot)

Is it at the beginning, throughout or at the end of the stream?

How often do you pass water? (frequency)

Any change in the amount? (anuria)

Any burning sensation with passing water? (dysuria)

On feeling to pass water, do you have to go at once? (urgency)

On wanting to pass water, is there delay before you start? (hesitancy)

Do you ever pass water when you don't want to? (incontinence)

Do you feel the bladder is not empty after passing water? (strangury)

Do you have tummy pain?

Pain in water pipe? (penis)

Pain in loin? (calculus)

Any lump in the tummy?

Any weight loss, tiredness, loss of appetite and night sweats?

Have you ever passed a stone before?

Any temperature?

Any discharge from the penis?

Any trauma to the tummy?

Did you have similar conditions in the past?

Do you have any bleeding from other sites?

Do you have any illness? (hypertension, DM or bleeding disorder, recurrent UTI)

Past-surgical history?

Do you take any medication? (Warfarin or aspirin)

Any family history of kidney problems or any other illnesses as bleeding disorders? (malignancy?)

Do you smoke?

Do you drink?

What is your job? Dye or rubber industry?

Did you travel abroad? (schistosomiasis)

Did you eat beetroot?"

Explain that you need to examine him and to run some tests and later tell him what is wrong with him.

"Is everything clear? Have you got any questions?

Thank you very much for your co-operation."

D/D

Renal stones

UTI

—

Schistosomiasis, terminal haematuria, travel abroad
Bladder carcinoma
Trauma
Prostate carcinoma
Coagulation disorder

RIGHT UPPER QUADRANT PAIN OF THE ABDOMEN

Greet, introduce yourself, identify, acknowledge and ask for consent.

"Could you describe the pain for me please?

It started suddenly or gradually?

Could you tell me where exactly the pain is?

How long it's been there? How severe it is?

Have you had any similar condition in the past?

How does it feel like?

Is it intermittent or is it constant and getting worse?

Is it there all the time or it come and goes?

Does it go anywhere?"

Anything makes it worse?

"Eating fatty meal or fried food?

Hunger?

Stress?

Breathing in?

Coughing?"

Anything make it better?

"Lying down or rolling around.

Medication?"

Associations

"How is your appetite? What kind of diet you eat?

Feeling sick? (nausea)

Being sick? (vomiting)

Any change in the bowel habit?

Any change in the colour of the motions? (blood)

Any recent temperature? Any rigor?

Chest pain, cough, SOB, phlegm +/- blood, wheeze?

Passing water more than usual? Any burning sensation while passing water? Any change in the colour of urine?

Night sweating?

Any weight loss?

Any lump in your tummy?

Any change in the colour of the skin or eyes?

Any itching of the skin? Any tiredness?

Have you had any recent blood transfusion?

Any recent chest trauma?

Have you travelled abroad recently?"

Past-medical history?

Past-surgical history?

On *any medications*?

Family history of similar conditions?

Social history

Alcohol? Occupation? Smoking?

"Thank you very much for your co-operation."

INTUSSUCEPTION

Greet, introduce yourself and identify the mother and her baby.

"I understand that your child is not feeling well. I need to ask you few questions about his condition. Is that OK to start with? (2 months to 2 yrs)

"Could you please tell me what has happened to him?

How long has he been crying?

Is he crying all the time or with periods of rest?

Does he draw the legs to the tummy? (sign of pain)

Pallor during the episode especially around the mouth?

How is his feeding?

Did you introduce any new type of food?

Has he been sick? (vomitting, billious/non-billious)

Did you notice any lump (sausage-shaped) in his tummy? Any visible movement?

How many times did he open his bowel?

Any changes in the stool consistency? Any changes in the colour? (red current jelly stool)

Does he seem to be dry? His mouth, tongue? Is he crying without tears? (dehydrated)

Does he have any temperature?

Any rash? Have you applied a glass to the rash?

How is his water works?

Is he active, tired or sleepy?

How is his breathing?

Is it the first time he has this?

Any illness apart from that?

On any medication?

Any family history of bowel disease or other diseases?"

"Well Ms.........., from what you have said, it seems that your child has what we call intussusception, it is a condition where a part of your child's bowel gets folded inside the another, just like my sleeves.

So first I need to examine him and then we need to run some tests.

The important one is what we call barium enema where we put a very thin tube into the back passage of your child and push a material which will make the condition appear on X-ray and in most cases it will treat the problem by unfolding the folded part.

In a very small number of patients this might fail to unfold the folded part, so we might have to do an operation which will allow us to look at the part of bowel and if it was still healthy we return it back to its proper position and if not, we will cut the unhealthy part and rejoin the ends of the bowel."

"Is everything is clear? Any questions?"

"Thank you very much for your co-operation."

NEEDLESTICK INJURY

Greet, introduce yourself and identify the mother and the child.

"I understand that you are worried as your child has pricked himself with a needle. I need to ask you a few questions about what has happened. Is that OK?

Could you please tell me more about what has happened?

How old is your boy?

When did this happen?

Were you with him? (If no, anybody else witnessed the incident?)

Did he bleed after that?

Did you clean the area?

Did you bring the needle with you?

Was the needle clean or dirty?

Do you know whom the needle belongs to? (Is he healthy or has he got hepatitis or HIV? or where has he found it?)

What about his immunization, is it complete?

When did he last have his tetanus immunization?"

"Well Mrs ...., there are a few things we need to do.

We'll dispose the needle for you.

The boy needs a blood test to check his hepatitis status.

We'll then give him the first dose of the vaccine.

He'll need two further boosters at 1st and 2nd month, which he should get from his GP.

He'll also need another blood test after the vaccination.

Regarding the risk of HIV, I can reassure you that the risk is very small.

I'll write to his GP about what needs to be done, it's important that the boy receives the full course of the immunization."

Assure her that it is a needlestick injury that occured in a park and therefore risk of viral infection is very less as a virus cannot survive in external environment for long time.

"Is everything is clear? Have you got any questions?"

"Thank you very much for your co-operation."

DIABETESE (CHILD)

Greet, introduce yourself and identify the mother and her child.

"I understand that your child is feeling a bit unwell.

I need to ask you a few questions about her condition.

Is that OK?

Could you tell me please what has happened to her?

When did you notice that she passed water more than usual?

Is it the first time she has this?

How many times does she pass water within a day?

Was it mainly at day or at night? (nocturnal enerusis)

Is it just increase in frequency or it is also increase in the amount of urine?

Any change in the colour of urine?

Any burning sensation while passing water?

Does she drink water more than usual?

Wakes up at night to drink water?

Does she seem to have dry mouth?

Does she cry without tears?

Does she seem to be sleepy?

Does she seem to be tired?

Has she lost weight recently?

How is her appetite?

Any tummy pain?

Any change in vision?

Does she seem to be feverish?
Any recurrent urinary infection?
Any whitish discharge or itch from down below?
Any injury to the head?
Meningitis?
Does she have any illness?
Any frequent loose motions?
Similar illness in the past?
Has she had full vaccinations?
Is she on any medication?
Any family history of DM?
Any other disease?"
"Have you got any questions to ask me?"
"Thank you very much for your co-operation."

MORPHINE ADDICTION

Greet, introduce, identify, acknowledge and ask for consent.

"For how long you have this?

Is it the first time or you had this before?

Anything that brings it on?"

Other complaints

"Allergy? (excessive sneezing, fever, sore throat, nasal obstruction).

Any medical illness?

On any medication? (pills, beta-blockers, NSAIDs, nasal decongestants, (rhinitis medicamentosa)

Do you smoke?

Do you drink alcohol?

Would you mind if I asked you a few personal questions? (ensure confidentiality)

Do you take anything else to enhance your mood?

Do you inject any drug?

How long have you been using this drug?

How often do you use it?

How many times in a day?

What happens if you stop taking it?

How do you use drugs? (injection or sniffing)

Where do you usually use drugs? How do you get your supply?

Do you share needles?

Do you have a partner?

Does s/he use drugs?

How do you finance your drugs? How much you spend on it?

Any problems at home/at work/with law?"

"Well Mr......................, drugs can cause many problems and can affect health. Do you have any idea about those harmful effects?"

Complications

Feeling sick and being sick.

Constipation.

Sleepiness.

It affects breathing and in high doses stops it.

Problems in vision.

Difficulty in passing water.

While using the drug for a long time, you get what we call *dependence* (that is when you do not use the drug you get irritable and feel craving for it and you get:

- Running nose.
- Running eyes.
- Tummy pain.
- Loose motions.
- Yawning.
- Disturbed sleep.
- Muscle pain.

Problems of injections: If a drug user *shares needles*, he may catch diseases such as AIDS, liver disease, chest infection and infection of the heart lining.

Using drugs can cause *financial problems and problems with the law*.

"Have you considered cutting down on morphine?

I can refer you to one of my colleagues who is specialised in that area to help you in cutting down.

And here are some leaflets about groups that are helping people who want to cut down drugs.

Have you got any questions to ask?

Is everything is clear?"

"Thank you very much for your co-operation.

I'm going to refer you to needle exchange programme, it may help you."

DEPRESSION

"Mrs. Smith, you look very concerned about something, can you tell me what is in your mind?"

If the patient is not responding to your initial question, you may repeat:

"Mrs Smith, when one is feeling low they feel better if they share their thoughts with the doctor, who will be able to help. I understand that you lost your husband a few months ago and this has been a devastating blow to you. Is there anything I can help you with?"

Introduce yourself and ask for consent by saying "I understand that ycu are finding life a bit difficult, Could you tell me what has been going on?".

Onset

Does the patient have insight to his/her complaint?

"How do you feel in yourself? Do you feel low?"

Ask for the symptoms of depression:

"Do you feel tired?"

SAWEMAIL

"How is your sleep?

Do you cry often?

Do you enjoy things you used to enjoy before?

How is your appetite?

Have you lost weight?"

Special questions

"Do you have any concerns about your health?

Do you think live is worth living nowadays?

Did you have any thoughts about harming yourself?

Or planned for that? Or attempted to do that?" (If yes, ask about what stopped him/her to do so? Did s/he try to leave any notice? "Do you think you may try it in future?"

Ask about symptoms of psychosis.

Risk factors - Age?

Premorbid personality

"How have you been feeling in yourself?"

Birth, growth and development

Childhood?

Friends and socialisation?

School?

Hobbies?

Past-psychiatric history

"Does anyone in your family suffer from a psychiatric illness, or mood problems?"

"Have you been feeling low before?"

If female:

"Do you suffer from PMT?"

Social History

Partner?

Relation with the partner?

"Do you feel any support from your family and friends? Feeling isolated?

Are you working? Having stress with your job?

Drinking alcohol? Which kind? How much?

Smoking?"

EPILEPSY

Introduction.

Ask the patient about:

Age?

Duration and frequency of the symptoms?

Establish the characteristics of the funny turns.

"What brings it on? (TV, sleep or trauma)

Any strange feelings before the attack?

Do you remember anything about the attack?

Anyone witnessed the attack? What did s/he said about it?

Didn't s/he mention anything about shaking your limbs or tongue biting?

Wetting yourself? Flushing of your face? Shaking of your limbs?

How did you feel after the attack? (headache, drowsiness and any injury)

Any similar attacks before?"

Exclude other neurological deficits + infection:

Headache

Fever?

"When you were fit-free, have you got any headaches?

Any change in speech?

Any visual or hearing loss?

Any dizziness?

Any weakness in the limbs?
Any loss of feeling in the limbs?"

Past-medical history

"Any history of:
Head injury?
Fever fits during childhood?
DM?
Hypertension?
Renal diseases?
Liver diseases?"

Medications

"On any medication?
Have you been taking any medication in the past?
On any recreational drugs?"

Family History

"Anyone in your family or relatives has similar conditions?" (epilepsy)

Social History

"What is your job?
Do you have any stress at work or at home?
Any sleep deprivation?
Watching TV frequently?
Smoking?
Drinking alcohol?"

CHILD ABUSE

Greet, introduce yourself and identify the mother.

Take a short history about the mechanism of the injury by asking: "Could you tell me what happened to the child?"

When?

Where?

How?

Anybody witnessed what happened?

Where were you at that time?

What did you do to help him?

Why?

Why delay in bringing the child to medical attention?

Has any injuries in the past? (head injury, spinal injury (cane, belts or rods), bruises over fingertips, on ribs and marks of cigarette burns).

Do you breast-feed or bottle-feed him?

How many children do you have?

Did they suffer any injury recently?"

Ask for permission of asking a few personal questions.

"I am duty bound to ask you a few questions.

Are you married?

Did you plan for this pregnancy?

Any problems during pregnancy?

Any problems after pregnancy?

Are you still living with your husband?

Or do you live together?

What are your jobs? Any financial problems?

Any history of taking alcohol or drugs to enhance your mood?"

R/o osteogenesis imperfecta, repeated multiple fracture, deafness, dwarfism.

Family history:

"Any sibling rivalry?"

Differential Diagnosis?

1. Osteogenesis imperfecta.
2. Mongolian blue-spots.
3. Battered baby syndrome or child abuse.

Points that make you suspicious:

1. Strange and unreliable history of injury.
2. Inappropriate injury to age.
3. Continuously changing history.
4. Vague history/ lacking details.
5. Delay in seeking medical attention.
6. Frequent AandE attendance.
7. Not enough food, clothing or shelter.
8. Leaving the child in unsafe place.
9. Frequent school absence.

Common Injuries:

1. Cuts, bruises.
2. Burns.

3. Fractures.
4. Hunger or thirst.
5. Frequent rash.
6. Fear.
7. Shyness.
8. Learning difficulties.

"With the details you have given, it doesn't really explain the nature of injury the child has sustained.

We are not blaming anyone but we are trying to do best for the child.

We might have to involve other department to help everyone."

HEADACHE / HISTORY

Greet, introduce yourself and identify the patient.

"I understand that you have headache. I need to ask you few a questions about your condition. Is that OK?".

"Could you tell me more about your headache?

How long have you had that headache? Or when did it start?

Is it similar to, or different from, the previous headaches?

Where it hurts exactly? (generalized or localized)

Did it come suddenly or gradually? (sudden: SAH, meningitis and migraine; insidious: ICP and migraine)

Can you tell me how it feels like? How sever it is: Dull, sharp or throbbing?

Does it go anywhere?

Does anything make it worse? (like early morning wakening, after lying down, straining at stool, coughing, laughing or combing your hair and eating)

Anything makes it better? (like medications as paracetamol, aspirin, NSAIDs or opiates)

Does anything seem to bring on the headache?" (stress, OCP, foods wine or alcohol)

Associated features

"Any strange feelings before the headache? (spots or flashing light)

Do you feel sick/been sick?

Does light or noise irritate you?

High temperature?

Do you feel any pain in your neck or difficulty to move your neck? Any rash?

Sore throat/cough/sinusitis/earache?

Lethargy and malaise? Weight loss?"

Fits

"Any problems with your vision? (blindness or double vision).

Do you feel weakness in your limbs?

Have you lost feelings in your limbs?

Were you aware all time? Did you feel sleepy?

Did you notice any change in your speech?

Any recent trauma to your head?"

Past-medical history

"Any chronic illness (hypertension, migraine, epilepsy)

Past surgery? (shunt)

On any medication? OCP?

Family history: Any similar condition in your family?

Social history: Any stress at job or at home?

Drinking alcohol?

Smoking?"

"Do you have any questions to ask me? Is everything clear?"

"Thank you very much for your co-operation."

D/D

Migraine

Aura

Recurrent episode

Family history

Relation to the precipitating factor (chocolate, dairy food, coffee, etc.)

Meningitis

Fever

Rash

Neck stiffness

ICSOL

Early morning headache

Projectile vomitting

Seizure

SAH

Sudden onset

Blow at the back of neck

Excrutiating

Sickness

Temporal arteritis

Scalp tenderness

Facial pain

Glaucoma—blurring of vision
OCP's- Benign intracranial HTN
Stress- tight band like
Refraction error
Sinusitis

COUNSELLING

CHANGING LIFE STYLE, MI

Introduction

"Good morning Mr. Brown, I am Dr ...., I am the SHO in medicine."

"You remember that you came a few days ago with sudden chest pain.

You are coming along very nicely and you are ready to go home tomorrow.

I think it would be a good idea if we have a little chat before going home.

I would like to give you advice on what to do and what not do from now on, and more importantly answer your entire question.

The tests showed that you had a heart attack. This is a condition where one of the vessels, which supply blood to the heart, becomes blocked by a clot. That area is damaged and is replaced by a scar in 4–6 weeks time.

This process takes from days to weeks and it is better not to put a great strain on the heart at this time. Within 2–3 months at most the hearts of many patients are functioning just about as well as before the attack."

Life Style

"Apart from medication, which I'll talk to you about later, there are some points about a little change of your life style."

Work

"You have to get some rest in home initially for 4–6 weeks,

You can gradually do some simple house hold work when you feel upto it after a couple of weeks but you shouldn't do any heavy lifting.

You can go back to work in 4–12 weeks depending on the type of work."

Diet

"It would be a good idea if you consider reducing your weight and avoid saturated fat especially high fat diary products, butter, fatty meal, coconut oil, fried meat, especially red meat.

You can eat more fresh fruit and vegetables, chicken (without skin), fish, skimmed and semi-skimmed milks, grill, and don't fry.

Cut down on alcohol, stop smoking all together."

Exercise

"You can start exercise gently and increase it with time.

Try to avoid walking in cold winds and climbing up steep hills.

About sports, you can take up golf, cycling, swimming, and bedside walking:

However, avoid sports with vigorous exercise as squash and weight-lifting."

Smoking

"You should give up smoking as it increases the risk of recurrent attacks."

Alcohol

"1 or 2 glasses of wine or ½–1 pint of beer or one measure of spirit does not affect the heart but more than this may give harm to the heart."

Sexual intercourse

"It increases the work of the heart and in some people causes chest pain or shortness of breath.

But in majority of cases, sexual activity can be resumed as soon as you are able to take other forms of moderate exercise as walking upstairs without symptoms.

GTN tablet before intercourse can help but you should give up immediately if you get chest pain."

Driving

"You can start after 4 weeks and it is better if you try short runs in the neighborhood accompanied by a friend.

Inform your driving license authority."

Stress

"It would be a good idea if you take up relaxation therapy and avoid stressful condition as much as you can."

Avoid air travel for six weeks.

Follow up

Base line inv. like

FBC

Blood sugar

Lipid profile

Treadmill test: Patient to undergo treatment test after six weeks.

If strainis +ve then *coronary angiogram* and review after the result.

Involve cardiac rehabilitation nurse.

Q. Can I have another heart attack?

"When you come back to clinic, we will do some investigation. If the results are fine, then taking your medication and changing your life style will decrease the chance of another heart attack. One cannot confirm that you will not have another heart attack."

Q. What is an angiogram?

"It is a special investigation in which a dye is injected in your vein and some X-ray is taken as the dye goes through coronary vessels, which supply blood to heart. This allows us to see if there is any blockage or narrowing of coronary vessels. It is road map of heart vessels."

AFTER MI, ADVICE MEDICATIONS

Introduction

"Good afternoon Mr. Smith, my name is Dr............... and I am the SHO in medicine." (shake hands)

"Now you are feeling much better, and you are ready to go home today.

I would like to explain you about your medication before you go home.

I will also try to answer all your questions.

Even before I start, I would like to emphasize that you should take all your medication everyday without fail and you shouldn't stop any medication without medical advice even if you are feeling well.

If you think any medicine does not suit you, you should call your doctor and take advice."

Beta-blocker

"This is *atenolol*. It prevents chest pain and helps in prevention of further attacks.

You should take one tablet everyday. Swallow one tablet with a glass of water.

It is a long-term treatment (usually for 2–3 years). Please do not stop taking this medication suddenly, because this may cause the pain to worsen and will affect your condition.

This medication sometimes causes side effects like slowing of heart rate and lowering of BP in some people, headache, sleepiness, bad dreams, dizziness, light headedness, shortness of breath, wheeze, slow pulse, skin rash, dry eye, tiredness, cold hands and feet, and impotence.

I will have to emphasize that these do not occur in every person.

You should not take this tablet if you have a poor blood circulation or asthma."

Aspirin

"This is *aspirin.*

You should take it once a day with a glass of water, sometime it causes irritation of stomach, and to prevent this it should be taken after meal (on full stomach).

This is a long-term treatment.

This drug thins your blood and prevents blockage of the blood vessels of the heart, which may result in another heart attack.

The side effects are mainly stomach irritation then it might cause tummy pain, blackish discoloration of stool, other unusual bleeding, and not all people have these.

If you notice any of these features or if you notice any bleeding, you should contact your doctor immediately."

Glycerol Trinitrate

"This is *GTN*.

You should take it in case if you have chest pain. Also, you can take before exercise, it will increase your exercise limit.

Put one tablet under your tongue and wait till it dissolves in your mouth. If the pain doesn't go, you can take another tablet (upto a total 1 mg),

Don't swallow, it acts by dilating arteries.

Side effects include headache, flushing, dizziness, especially, when you get up suddenly (postural hypotension).

These side effects are usually short term. If you notice any of these, consult your doctor.

I would like to assure you that it is not habit-forming or addictive and it has very short expiry date."

"Do you have any question about your medication?

Thank you." (Also thank the examiner.)

Q. Is it possible that these drugs will be stopped in future?

If you don't have any side effects, it is unlikely that they will be stopped.

Q. Will these tablets affect my sex life?

"Sex is safe if you can climb two flights of stairs without any breathlessness or chest pain.

Have GTN spray/tablet if angina is a problem.

Sex is safe if after a goodnight sleep.

Avoid sex after a hot bath or a full stomach."

CONSENT HERNIORRHAPHY AND POST-OP ADVICE

Greet, introduce yourself and identify the patient.

"I need to have a word with you about your hernia and possibility of surgical treatment and to take your consent about the operation. Is that OK ?"

"Do you have any idea about what herniorrhaphy is?

Hernia is a defect in the tummy wall through which the contents of the tummy try to come out when you cough or strain.

The predisposing factors that can lead to hernia are:

Lifting heavy objects,

straining as in constipation,

being overweight,

chronic cough,

and previous abdominal surgery.

If we don't treat it, it grows and gets twisted and become irreducible, thereby reducing or even cutting the blood supply of that portion of the bowel and causing the death of the tissue which will be 'life-threatening'.

The surgical treatment may be done laparoscopically (key hole surgery) or by formal surgery.

You must not eat or drink after midnight the day before the operation (however, it is important that he takes his morning medication with a sip of water).

The operation will take about 1 hour.

You will have either general anaesthesia where you will be put to sleep and then you wake up after the operation; or you will have spinal anaesthesia where you will be given an injection into the backbone and you will feel numb from waist below.

We are going to make a cut of 2 inches length in the area of the hernia.

We return the contents of the tummy as gut and covering back into their proper position and the weak area is repaired either by using a synthetic mesh, darning by nylon, or repositioning of the muscles.

You will wake up from general anaesthesia in the recovery area and once you wake up, you will be taken back to the ward.

You will probably feel sleepy for a couple of hours.

You may feel sick, get headache or sore throat.

This will pass but be sure to inform the nursing staff should this become worse.

As any operation, this may have some complications.

Not everyone will have these but we are bound to tell these to everyone.

Wound infection, which is going to be treated by appropriate antibiotics.

Bleeding (that is going to be treated by finding its source and stopping it) and collection of the blood in the area that is going to be drained.

There is a low risk of failure of the operation or *recurrence* (10%).

You may feel *pain after the operation* and that is going to be controlled adequately by strong painkillers (Diclofenac IM or IVI 10 mg qqh, Morphine SC or IM 10 mg qqh or PCA device (need for oxygen with it)).

There is a very low risk of *infertility* (<1%) and as you are in good hands, we will find the structures related to fertility and put them away from the work field.

Urine retention, chest infection, and clots in the leg and the lungs.

You will remain in hospital for 1–2 days after the operation (*if GA is used*) or you will be sent home with analgesia on the same day of the operation (*if SA is used*). You will need to arrange for someone to pick you up and drive you home on the evening of the operation.

If dissolvable stitches are used, they will dissolve by themselves within 7 days; but if external (non-dissolvable) stitches are used, they will need to be removed in 5–7 days.

Lifestyle

You need to have *rest* for 1 week after the operation.

You could be back to *light or desk work* after 2 weeks but *manual work* after 3 months (avoid excessive straining or lifting of heavy weights).

Drive after 1–2 weeks or when it is comfortable.

Sex as soon as comfortable.

Diet have a lot of vegetables and fruits.

Smoking is better to be stopped.

You may need to return to outpatient clinic 6 weeks after the operation.

The operation will be done by Dr...................... and he will have the overall responsibility for the treatment.

You are free to change your mind anytime about your decision and you have a full right to seek a second opinion.

I know it must be an anxious moment for you and I am sorry to give you so much information, it's important that you understand what we are planning for you.

Don't worry, you are in good hands and we will do our best for you.

Is everything clear to you?

Do you have any questions to ask me?"

"This is the consent form for the operation, would you mind reading it.

If you agree about the operation, would you mind writing your name, signing and dating the form where indicated please?"

"Thank you very much for your co-operation."

POST-MORTEM EXAMINATION

Greet, introduce yourself and identify the lady.

"I've got a rather delicate matter to discuss with you,

It is about your sister.

You know she was coming along very well after the operation, but she suddenly had a chest pain and we tried to save her life.

We did everything we could but she passed away.

I'm so sorry about that .... Do you need a cup of water or shall I call a friend of yours.

I'm so sorry for your sister...................... I understand that it's really hard to come to term with...................... Please accept my sympathy and condolences and convey them to the rest of the family.

We and the Coroner need to know the cause of the death and its importance is to see whether it's familial and to prevent future losses and save lives.

We need to do what we call 'post-mortem examination'. Do you know anything about it?

It's just like a surgical operation done by special doctors.

We are going to look inside her body and take samples of tissues from organs and fluids to examine them in order to know the cause of the death. They will be treated with dignity and respect and we wouldn't misuse them.

We are not going to take any organ out and we wouldn't disturb the body.

Is that alright?".

If the answer for the previous question was 'No', then say : "Our feeling is natural and most people will feel exactly the same, but I'd like you to think about it and discuss it with the rest of the family members. At the end it's entirely up to you."

"Have you got any other concerns in regard to your sister's death?

Feel free to ask any time.

Could you please read this consent form and when you agree, sign it and date it in below?"

"Thank you very much for your co-operation."

Will it disfigure the body?

"This examination is done by experienced hospital pathologists and it goes like a surgical procedure with little disfigurement, if any.

Dignity and respect will be the priority.

The pathologist examines only the precise organs requested. No organs will be removed or biopsied without your knowledge and written permission."

Will be there many people watching this?

"Usually only medical students are there, if you don't want them to be there, it can be done."

Can I refuse?

"Certainly, but we may miss the cause of the death."

Did she suffer pain?

"When she had the chest pain, we gave her analgesics along with the treatment needed and I can assure you that she passed away peacefully."

"The whole process doesn't take more than a few hours. If you are prepared for a funeral you can carry on with your preparation.

Do you want to know what has happened or what will happen next?"

UPPER GI ENDOSCOPY

Greet, introduce yourself and identify the patient.

Ascertain how much does the patient know about the procedure?

"An endoscope is a thin, flexible tube which is as thin as a finger (1 cm in diameter) with a tiny camera attached to its end and is passed down through the gullet down to your stomach.

An experienced doctor performs it.

The whole procedure takes about 15–20 minutes.

We are going to numb your throat by a local anaesthetic spray.

Sedation can be given but not general anaesthesia.

You can take your breakfast and we are going to do it at afternoon (6–8 hour fasting before the procedure).

The doctor is going to look at your gullet and stomach and upper part of your bowel and he might take tiny pieces of tissue from your stomach to examine it under microscope to find out the exact nature of the problem.

It may be uncomfortable but not painful.

You have to stay at hospital for at least 1 hour after the procedure. (You should avoid eating and drinking for 1 hour.)

You can go home on the same day but you should not drive because the anaesthesia makes you drowsy."

Side effects

Common

Sore throat.

Drowsiness from the sedation used.

Uncommon

Slight bleeding from the sites when tissue has been taken.

Oesophageal tear: If it was small, it will spontaneously heal by itself, if it was large it may lead to collection of air in the chest wall (pneumomediastinum, which may require surgery).

Infection of the structures surrounding your gullet (mediastinitis, treatment is by antibiotics).

Ask the patient about any concerns.

"Here is the consent form, can you please read it, sign it and date it?"

"Thank you very much for your co-operation."

ECTOPIC PREGNANCY, LAPAROSCOPY

Introduction, ...

"Now, we have had a good look at your tests that we run. And according to the results of the tests, the examination, and what you complained of, there is a high possibility that you have what we call ectopic pregnancy, that is a pregnancy outside your womb.

This can be in the tubes between your womb and ovaries as in most cases, or at the ovary or inside the tummy, which is very rare. And since the pregnancy is not in the usual place, it cannot continue to term.

In addition, it may bleed suddenly or even cause damage to the tube, which could cause you some harm.

To avoid these problems, we have first to be sure that you have ectopic pregnancy and the best way to do this is by laparoscope.

That is the procedure by which we insert a tube with lenses within a small incision in your tummy, after we put you into sleep. So we could look at your womb and tubes.

And to treat the condition, there are two ways.

Either by laparoscopy, where we could either inject a medication called methotrexate or remove the pregnancy by incision.

The second way to deal with this condition is by operation to remove the pregnancy. And in either ways of treatment we will try to conserve the tube, but if it is damaged by this condition, then the only way to deal with it, is to remove the tube."

"Is everything clear or do you want me to repeat anything for you?

Are there any questions that you would like to ask me?"

"You will remain for 2-3 days in the hospital.

You can return to work after 6 weeks (sick leave).

The doctor will make 2 incisions, one just below the navel and the second above the bikini line."

PRE-ECLAMPSIA

Greet, introduce, identify, acknowledge and ask for consent.

"I understand that you are insisting to go home to take care of your daughter.

I need to have a few words with you about your condition and we'll talk about your daughter as well. Is that alright?"

"Well, as we examined you and according to the results of the tests we have done for you, you have a condition what we call pregnancy-induced hypertension.

It's high blood pressure during pregnancy with some other changes and in these cases we admit the patient to the hospital so that we can give her the treatment she needs and do all the tests needed to keep an eye on her.

The period needed to remain in hospital depends on the condition of the patient and her response to the treatment.

In some cases if the patient doesn't respond to the treatment, we may even need to end the pregnancy earlier and that is the important reason to remain in hospital, as we can take care of the mother and there is a doctor who will take care of the baby.

In addition, in some severe cases the mother might develop fits.

So in the hospital we can act quickly to manage her condition, otherwise that will pose a great threat on your life and your baby's life without urgent treatment."

Tell her that it's a must to stay at hospital until she recovers or the pregnancy is terminated.

"Now let us talk about your daughter.

Have you got a partner to look after her?

Can you get help from your mother or sister?

Have you got relatives to look after her?"

If the answer for all the above questions is 'No', then say that "we can arrange for social services to look after her during that period."

"Is everything clear? Have you got any questions?"

"Thank you very much for your co-operation."

BABY BLUES, POST-NATAL DEPRESSION

In case of Baby Blues

(It is the commonest condition in first 3-4 days after delivery and lasts for a few days.)

"Well, Mrs ...., what you have is what we call *Baby Blues*, it is a very common condition and occurs in more than one of every 2 mothers after delivery.

What you need is just rest, try to have more sleep, eat healthy food with lot of vegetables and fruit and try to get out with your partner. Have fun with him and you will be OK in a few days. And as for the child, the doctor has seen and said that nothing is wrong with him, so there is nothing to worry about, and you can contact us at any time you feel the need to."

In case of Post-Natal Depression

(It is the commonest condition in the first month up to 6 months.)

"Well Mrs ...., what you have is what we call post-natal depression. We will refer you to another department in this hospital; they will give you some medication.

You will get better, but it takes some time and meanwhile we will arrange support for you.

It is a common condition and can be treated, so don't worry about it."

CIN III. EXPLAIN COLPOSCOPY AND BIOPSY

Introduce yourself.

Break bad news by reassuring the patient that abnormal cervical smear is very common in women 1/12, it doesn't mean cancer, it's just a warning sign.

"For this reason, we have to do another investigation, what we call *colposcopy* by which we can identify the exact nature of the change.

By this stage, the treatment is available and it's simple and virtually 100% effective."

Colposcopy

"It's a day case procedure.

It lasts 15 minutes.

It is not painful but you may feel uncomfortable.

There may be a little or no effect on fertility.

There is no risk of having miscarriages."

Post-procedure advice

"Bleeding and discharge for 5 days

Avoid intercourse for 5 days.

Is there anything that is not clear to you?

What is next when the results come?"

If the results were normal, the patient should be followed up after 6 months by having another cervical smear and colposcopy, if the results of which were normal, consider following up the patient yearly in the next 4–5 years.

TERMINATION OF PREGNANCY (TOP)

Greet, introduce, identify, acknowledge and ask for consent.

"I understand that you want to terminate your pregnancy. Is that alright to talk about that?

How old are you?

Could you tell me why do you want to terminate your pregnancy?

Have you thought about other options to avoid this decision?

Help from family or adoption.

Remember that you will live with that decision for life.

Have you got a partner?

Does he know about your decision?"

Periods

"When was your last period?

Were they regular?"

Management

US (to examine for the state of pregnancy)

Blood grouping (is she RhD-ve, anti-D required?)

Swab from the front passage (chlamydia).

Prophylactic tetracycline is given.

TOP

If in the *first trimester*, the commonest method is D and C or D and V

If in the *second trimester*

(Induce labour)

Prostaglandins.

IV Oxytocin.

Complications of TOP

Bleeding.

Infection.

Damage to the womb and its neck.

It may affect chance of future pregnancy.

It may increase the chance of miscarriage.

Psychiatric problems.

1:100,000 risk of death.

"We can give you contraception to use at the day of TOP if you want.

Any questions?

Here is the consent form, can you sign it please?

Thank you very much for your co-operation."

HRT COUNSELLING?

Introduce yourself.

Describe menopause if needed.

Effects of the lack of oestrogen on the body :

1. Brain
   a. Mood changes.
   b. Lack of concern.
   c. Forgetfullness.
2. Bone
   a. Brittleness.
   b. Falls.
   c. Fractures.
3. Skin
   a. Hot flushes.
   b. Dry skin.
   c. Easily bruised.
   d. Vaginal symptoms.

Forms of HRT

1. Tablets (taken daily)
2. Gels (used daily)
3. Patches (twice a week)
4. Cream and pessaries
5. Oestrogen-containging rings.

HRT cannot be used in

1. Liver diseases.
2. Ca breast.

3. Ca womb.
4. Vaginal bleeding of unknown cause.
5. Blood clotting disorders.

Side effects of HRT

1. It will increase the risk of Ca breast and womb, specially if used >10–15 years.
2. *Tabs*: Sickness, put on weight, mood changes and premenstrual syndrome.
3. *Patches*: Skin irritation.

NB.

1. Pessaries, creams and vaginal rings can be used without progesterone for intermittent use, otherwise, progesterone should be added to oestrogen with all types of HRT in those women who have wombs, especially when they are used continuously.

2. Oestrogen only HRT is used for those women who have undergone hysterectomy.

MESOTHILIOMA

Introduction.

"I would like to have a few words with you about your husband's condition.

As you know your husband came to us with shortness of breath and has been with us for some time.

We examined him and ran all the necessary investigations. I am sorry to have to tell you that he has a nasty growth in the lining of the lung that has already spread, so we cannot take it out by surgery.

I understand that this is not easy to come to terms with, but I can assure you that we will do our best to make the quality of his life better.

He may get some pain and fortunately we have many effective medicines to deal with pain.

First we start with Paractamol, which is given as 2 tablets 4 times daily, we may need to give him NSAIDs, such as Aspirin, Ibuprofen.

These may irritate the stomach and may cause some tummy pain so these should be taken with food.

And these drugs may cause some blood to appear in the stool.

We may combine these with weak opioids, such as dextropropoxyphene, and if pain is not controlled we can use strong opioids, such as morphine, which is effective.

There are side effects, such as feeling sick, being sick, sleepiness, constipation and respiratory depression.

However, we can adjust the dose of treatment, should these side effects occur."

"Another thing, that is, from time to time your husband may get shortness of breath because of fluid being collected in the lining of the lungs.

If he get this, you can bring him to the hospital so that we can take out some of the accumulated fluid to improve his breath.

Is everything clear?

Do you have any question?"

CA BREAST, DEPRESSED

Introduction.

"I would like to have a word with you about your condition. As far as I know, you have a nasty growth in your breast.

How do you feel in yourself now?

I understand that this is not easy to come to terms with, but I can assure you that with modern treatment thousands of lives have been saved and made comfortable.

Fortunately, we have a good management plan. First we have to do surgery. That is, we remove the growth together with your breast: This operation is called *mastectomy*.

This operation is done under general anaesthesia, where you will be put into sleep.

It is a major operation, after which you may feel unwell for a few days. There are chances of complications like bleeding, pain and infection.

And for minimising the chance of getting such complication we will give you medications.

You will probably be allowed up, the day after the operation.

You should remain in the hospital for 5–7 days.

And you can return to work in 6 weeks.

After the operation, we will give you a temporary breast form to wear under your bra until the site of operation heals completely, then we can arrange for a more lasting breast form.

Since mastectomy was introduced, this operation is carried out all over the world and women who underwent mastectomy are enjoying normal, useful and happy lives.

After thc operation you may need radiotherapy for 4–6 weeks daily in hospital; side effects are redness of skin, local hair loss and local effect.

We need to give you a type of medication called Tamoxifen that reduces the effect of female hormone called oestrogen or instead we may give you chemotherapy.

Chemotherapy is best for premenopausal cases.

Tamoxifen for postmenopausal cases.

You are not alone: It is a common condition which affects 1 in 12 women in the world."

STILLBIRTH

Introduction.

"How do you feel in yourself now?

I understand that it is not easy to come to term with, but you know it has happened to many people.

Do you want to see your baby, hold or take a photograph with him?

You can even take a lock of hair or palm prints if you want.

You can name him, and for funeral you can make a private one if you want, or the hospital can arrange a funeral for him.

I want to take a blood sample from you.

Also to take a swab from vagina and blood from the baby and send it for examination.

That would help us to know the cause of what has happened.

It would be so useful for us to know the cause of what has happened and to arrange for future pregnancy if we could send him for postmortem examination.

That is an operation-like examination.

This may help avoiding such a condition in future."

If she refuses, then ask her for permission to take a type of X-ray (MRI), and a sample of tissue for examination.

"I am going to give you a medication to decrease breast milk secretion, and we will give you an appointment to discuss future plans when the results of these tests come back.

We will give you a certificate of stillbirth that you need to take it to the Registrar of Birth and Death within 42 days.

I will give you the address of the local branch of bereavement counselling which might be useful for you.

It is preferable not to get pregnant in the next 6 months to 1 year."

HYPERTENSION

"Hello Mr ...., I am Dr .... and I am SHO in medicine. How are you feeling now?

I want to tell you about your blood pressure and also start some tablets for you. Is this OK with you?"

"As you know we measured your BP on a few occasions and every time it has been high. We have done a few tests to know if there is any cause for your hypertension.

All these tests have been negative.

What we think you have is *essential hypertension,* that is high blood pressure without any apparent cause.

This is a common problem and the cause is unknown; we can treat this with medications. I will also tell some life-style changes which will help.

Do you have any question before I proceed?"

Life style

"Do you smoke?"

If 'No', say "That's very good."

If 'Yes', say "You should stop smoking completely. I can suggest some help groups if you want."

Diet

"You should reduce salt intake and take a low fat diet.

Decrease your alcohol intake.

Avoid oily foods, take plenty of fruits and vegetables, no red meat, white meat (poultry) is fine. Fish is very good."

Weight

"What is your weight?"

If obese, say "You should reduce it."

Exercise

"Exercise is very helpful to decrease weight and keeps you fit."

Sex life

"As long as your blood pressure is under control, you should not have any problem with your sex life."

"Do you have any questions before I move to medications?"

Medication

"I have to emphasize that it is not a curable condition and you will need to take medication probably for the rest of your life.

You have to keep taking medicine even when you are feeling completely normal.

It normally takes a few days for the blood pressure to come down to normal. We will be keeping an eye on it and change your medication accordingly."

Thiazides

"This is the usual first choice drug.

It is the 'water tablet' and needs to be taken in the morning.

The side effects include impotence, lower blood pressure when you suddenly stand up and it can lower some of your salt."

Atenolol

"This tablet needs to be taken once a day.

It can slow your heart rate, cause impotence, cold peripheries and lethargy.

You should not take it if you have asthma and low circulation.

I have to emphasize that not everyone has these side effects.

If you have any, we can change your medication.

We will see you again in 4 weeks to see how your BP control is.

Do you have any question?"

PATIENT: "But I am feeling fine doctor, do I need to take the medicines?"

YOU: "It can affect your kidney, can give you heart attack, stroke and also visual impairment, if not treated."

COUNSELLING (PNEUMONIA)

"As you know you have come to us with some complain in your chest.

We did some test on you and the results are back you are suffering from a chest infection called pneumonia.

Do you know anything about it?

Pneumonia is nothing but infection of your lungs.

We need to run some more investigations to find out the actual bug causing it.

We will be giving you antibiotics till your infection subsides.

We would advise you to stay in hospital till this period, as we need to give directly in your blood.

I also advise you to take bed rest till you feel comfortable.

This is a very common thing, which many people get. You don't have to worry about it and you can go back to complete normal life after you recover.

Do you have any doubts regarding the condition?"

What are the complications?

"If not treated properly, it can become life-threatening and cause:

Abscess/empyema,

SOB,

Dehydration,

Pleural effusion,

Septicemia."

Can I go home now?

"You have to stay in hospital, as we have to give you medication intravenously.

If not treated properly, it can be life-threatening.

If you are dehydrated, we have to give you IV fluid.

If you have shortness of breath, we may consider giving you supplemental oxygen.

If you are getting more phlegm, we may have to go in for physiotherapy.

If left untreated, the infection might spread beyond lungs into body causing *septicaemia*

You might get pus in lung covering, which is known as *empyema*."

Can I take oral tablet?

"We would recommend the antibiotics directly into blood, as these are more effective than oral tablets.

We might change them later on oral tablet on advice of the microbiologist who is a specialist in controlling infection."

ASTHMA

Greet, introduce, identify, acknowledge and ask for consent.

"I have gone through your case notes and as you know you have a condition called *Asthma.*"

Do you know about this?

"Asthma is a condition in which the branches of wind-pipe in lung narrow down due to various causes and this causes difficulty in breathing common causes are exposure to allergens like pollen, dust, mite, etc., and infection."

General advice

"You should:

1. Avoid allergens, if known,
2. Keep a card with medication,
3. Take extra precaution to prevent chest infection, and
4. Start early treatment of infection.

It cannot be cured but can be controlled by using medications of two types:

1. Salbutamol
2. Beclamethasone

"I understand that you are feeling much better now and you are ready to go home.

I need to have a few words with you about the medications that you are going to take at home. Is that OK?".

"Have you got any idea about these medications (Becotide inhaler, Salbutamol inhaler and Prednisolone tablets)?

Have you used them before?"

Becotide inhaler

"It reduces inflammation of your airways and thus reducing their blockage. It should be used 2–4 times daily. It must be used regularly to obtain a maximum effect. There may be alleviation of your symptoms after the initiation of its use within 3–7 days but this will disappear soon. It may have some side effects as fungal infection of mouth and throat and hypersensitivity reaction to this medication which might occur with high doses. It is advised to wash your mouth after each use to decrease the risk of that infection.

Some patients may have glaucoma, cataract, weakness and tiredness or bone brittleness with long-term use of high doses. We are going to follow up regularly so as to give you a minimum dose required to control your symptoms."

Salbutamol inhaler

"It will relax the muscles of your windpipe hence reducing the risk of its blockage. It should be used according to the need (up to 3-4 times). Just like other medications, it may have some side effects, when it is used at a high dose, such as headache, trembling of the hands, heart racing, very rarely it might cause disturbance of the heart's electrical activity and disturbance of sleep and behaviour (in children). Rash, tiredness and weakness are other rare side effects which might occur. If you notice any of these side effects consult your doctor (paradoxical bronchospasm and tolerance)."

Prednisolone

"It has similar effects to Becotide on your windpipe. It is important to take this medication on full stomach.

Take 1 tablet everyday. It may have some side effects, but because it is used for a very short period, the chance of having these side effects is extremely slim. The side effects include irritation of the stomach, difficulty of digestion. Other side effects, which might occur with long-term use of high doses are fungal infection, muscle weakness, bone brittleness, menstrual irregularities, tiredness, sleep disturbance, change of vision and weight gain.

We are going to give you a steroid card and it's advised to take it with you always wherever you go and show it to anyone who treats you (nurse, dentist or pharmacist) and please try to contact your doctor immediately whenever you have any infection and try to make sure that the information on the card is kept up-to-date."

"Is everything clear? Have you got any questions to ask?"

"Thank you very much for your co-operation."

FEBRILE CONVULSION

Greet, introduce, identify, acknowledge and ask for consent.

Ask the child name and age from now on; address the child by his/her name, this will create good rapport.

"I understand that you are very worried about your child because s/he has got fits. I need to ask you a few questions and we'll talk about what to do next. Is that alright?"

Take a short history about the fits:

When?

What happened to the child?

Frequency?

Duration?

Which was the first event fever or fits?

Does it follow fever always?

Fever

Onset

Duration

Progression

How high?

***Febrile convulsion should be <3 fits and each lasting < 5 minutes.**

Continuous/intermittent

Aggravating / relieving factor

Fits

First attack/ recurrent

Generalised/focal

Describe the episode

Duration and how did it end

"Is she passing any water or biting the tongue after the attack.

Whether you saw the episode personally."

Immunization History

Exclude meningitis, and other infections as ear infection, sore throat, or chest infection and head injury.

Any family history of epilepsy/febrile convulsion, on any medication.

"Fever fits/ febrile convulsion are very common and present in 3% of children who get fever between 6 months and 5 years.

The reason is unknown in most of cases, but there is a genetic predisposition 10–20% cases, reassure the mother by saying "Your child isn't going to feel pain during the fits, don't worry s/he will be safe. What you have to do is to keep her/him safe during the fits, don't try to stop his/her movements and don't hold him tight."

Epilepsy subsequently?

"Febrile convulsion is a benign prognosis and there is very less chance <1% to develop epilepsy subsequently."

Management

Fever

"When s/he has high temperature, try to reduce it by • removing warm clothing, cooling environment, tepid sponging or by • Paracetamol 12 mg/kg, paracetamol syrup 120 mg/5 ml if temp doesn't settle down seek immediately."

Fits

"We will teach you how to give a medication called Diazepam through the back passage of your child (<3 years 5 mg, >3 years 10 mg) as a prophylaxis to the fits when your child has high fever. If the fit lasted > 5 minutes, call for an ambulance immediately get the child to A and E."

Talk about the small risk of getting epilepsy (3%) in future and 2% in siblings.

"Is everything clear? Have you got any questions?"

"Thank you very much for your co-operation."

MENINGITIS

"Is that Mrs .... ? This is Dr .... How can I help you?"

"How long he has been like this (feverish)? Have did you measure his temperature? How high it is? Any similar episodes in the past?

Any associated chills and sweating?

Are his hands or feet cold? (shock)

Any headache?

Any joint pain?

Is he active, walking, playing? Or drowsy and sleepy all the time?

Is he irritable and crying?

Any fits?

Is the child refusing food?

Has he been sick?

Did you notice he would shy away from light? Does he disliked bright light?

Can he move his head freely? Any pain when moving the neck?

Any skin rash? Does it blanch to pressure? (tell about the glass test)

Any tummy pain?

How is his water works? Any change in colour of the urine?

Has he had any recent infection?

Has he had any contact with other children at school or play area who have developed the same features?

How are your other children?

Has he been immunized regularly?"

"Well, Mrs......................., I need you to bring the child to hospital as soon as possible because from what you said it seems that your child has meningitis which needs to be treated as soon as possible, otherwise there will be the danger of losing your child. So please try to come to hospital as soon as possible. If you can't bring him, I'll send an ambulance to pick you up. Meanwhile try to isolate your child from the others, even yourself, because the infection is transmittable to others. Is that OK?"

"Is everything clear? Any questions?"

"Thanks, bye."

MENINGITIS OR URTI ?

Greet, introduce yourself and identify the mother.

"I can imagine how worried you are because you think your child might have meningitis, isn't it?

I can tell you for sure that it is not the case and I can reassure you he has not got meningitis.

You don't need to be worried because we examined the child and we found that he has no signs of meningitis and I'm going to explain to you why is that. Is that OK?

He has some fever and his temperature is 37.5 °C, which is mild fever (temperature), while in meningitis children will have a very high temperature.

A child with meningitis has a very severe headache whereas your child has just a mild headache and a patient with meningitis becomes very tired and sleepy while your child moves well around.

Besides, a child with meningitis can even develop fits, become sick many times and doesn't like food, and as you know your child has become sick once and he can eat.

Someone with meningitis usually dislikes light and shies away from it but your child can look nicely at light.

Also a child with meningitis finds it difficult to move his neck, which may be painful but your child can move his neck freely and with no problem.

Your child has no skin rash, which might occur in children with meningitis.

Besides, after examining your child we are pretty sure that he has what we call pharyngitis which is inflammation of the throat.

It is a good idea to be careful and keep a careful eye on him and as I have told there is nothing to worry about."

"Is everything is clear? Any questions to ask me please?"

"Thank you very much for your co-operation."

HIV POSITIVE

Greet, introduce, identify, acknowledge and ask for consent.

"I understand that you are here to know the results of your blood tests." I need to have a few words with you about this. Is that alright?"

"Before I tell you about what the result is, could you please tell me what do you think the result would be?"

If the answer was "HIV", then you would say "I'm afraid it is".

If the answer was "I don't know or could be an infection", then you say that "Well, at the beginning we thought about the same but I'm afraid it is not". The patient may ask "What do you mean by that doctor?" Your answer would be "I'm afraid to say that you have HIV in your body."

The patient will say "Ohhh my Godddd!!!.........."

You have to say "I understand it is really hard to come to term with ...."

"Do you want me to call any of your relatives or friends?"

"I can tell you that having the virus in your body does not mean that you have AIDS and in many cases it may take a very long time between having the virus in your body and until the AIDS disease manifests. (10–12 years)

Although, at present, there is no cure for this disease but there are a few medicines which may delay the onset of AIDS; medical field has made rapid progress and one can hope medicine for HIV will be available.

I can tell you for sure that this result will be strictly confidential.

We would like to do some more tests.

It will tell us at what stage the disease is."

Personal history: Ask for details like: Stable relationship, smoking, drinking, any recreational drugs, socio-economic status, friends and family support?

"It is very important to consider telling your partner about this and to bring her to have a health check up too if she wants to.

I understand it will be very much on you to digest all of these, but I need to tell you about few important precautions which you need to take.

It is very important to use condoms while you are having sex and to tell to the person who is going to have sex with you do not share needles.

It would be advised to consider cutting down on alcohol.

This infection can be transmitted by blood transfusion that is why it is advised to avoid giving blood to other people and not to donate organs.

It is up to you to inform your GP and your employer about this."

MINOCYCLINE, READ AN ARTICLE ABOUT THE SIDE EFFECTS

Greet, introduce yourself and identify the patient.

"I understand that you are worried about the side effects of the medication you take which is called Minocycline, because you've read an article about that. I need to talk to you about that medication. Is that OK?"

"Could you tell me what is written about its side effects? Well, I didn't read this article but I have read the original article in the *Lancet* from which it is taken."

"You need not get over-anxious about matters in media because as you know the newspapers tend to exaggerate things.

If you remember when we gave you this medication, we talked about the side effects.

And we said that it may make you feel sick or even been sick, it may cause having frequent loose motions, some skin rash, dizziness and giddiness.

These are the common side-effects and we know that this medication, in very few cases, might cause liver damage and that is why we take a tiny drop of blood from you every 6 months to monitor for any effect on the liver. As I've told you the media tends to take minor things and make major stories out of them.

In addition, you know that this is a new medication, so there might be some new side-effects that might appear as the time goes by, but we keep following any new side-effects that may occur and follow our patient up for that."

"Is everything clear? Have you got any questions to ask?"

"Thank you very much for your co-operation."

LAPAROSCOPIC CHOLECYSTECTOMY

Greet, introduce yourself and identify the patient.

"So you will have your gallbladder taken out by laparoscopy. Do you know anything about this procedure?

The procedure takes about 1–2 hours.

You will be asleep during the procedure (a GA is given).

The surgeon is going to make 4 small cuts (1 cm) in your tummy.

A tiny telescope-like instrument is passed through one of these cuts and the instruments which are used by the surgeon are passed through the other cuts.

We have to put what we call 'NG tube' through nostrils down to the stomach and another tube in your arm to give fluid to your blood.

Usually we use dissolvable (absorbable) stitches."

Advantages

"This procedure has many advantages over open surgery, which was used in the past:

Cuts are smaller and cause less upset to the body (open surgery cut is ~10 cm).

Muscles are not affected.

It is less painful.

You can return home and work quicker.

However, sometimes during the procedure conversion to open surgery is necessary."

Complications

"As any other surgical procedure, this operation may have some complications:

1. Infection of the wound is the most common complication and antibiotics are given to decrease this chance.
2. Bleeding: There may be some bleeding from the wound.
3. Pain at the wound site and often in the right shoulder tip (air inflation) for a day or two after the operation and you'll be given medication to relieve it.
4. Injury to the bile duct may happen during the procedure.
5. Blood clots may develop in the vein of the leg and to prevent this from happening you'll wear elastic stockings before, during and after the procedure, and you'll be encouraged to walk as soon as possible."

After the operation

"You'll be able to drink water after 4 hours.

You can start eating the day after the operation.

You may go home on the day after.

In general, you'll be kept in hospital until you are able to eat, drink and your pain is controlled."

After discharge

"1. *Diet:* Initially you should decrease fat in your diet.

2. *At work:* You are able to return to light work after 2 weeks.

3. *Driving and Sex:* You can start as soon as you don't have pain and is comfortable.

4. *Wound care:* You can bathe/shower as normal but avoid rubbing the wound or wearing tight clothes. That may irritate it.

5. Appointment after 6 weeks.

Pre-operative: You will observe fasting for 8 hrs before the operation."

LYMPHOMA, GOING TO PUT HER ON MORPHINE

Greet, introduce, identify, acknowledge and ask for verbal consent.

"I understand that you are here because you still have pain which couldn't be controlled by that medication ibuprofen. I need to have a few words with you about the new painkiller which we considered to give you. Is that OK?

"Well, the new medication is morphine. Have you got any idea about that medication?

Morphine has a very powerful effect on controlling pain, and we will start to give you one tablet every 4 hours until you get complete relief of pain.

Then we will change it to one tablet twice daily with the same dose of a longer-acting form of this medicine (sustained release with less side effects).

Apart from pain control, morphine has a very relieving effect on your mood.

In some cases, morphine cannot be taken by mouth, then we give it by muscle injection or injection into blood, or can be given underneath the skin injection by a syringe driver.

Just like any other medication, morphine has some side effects such as *feeling sick, being sick*. Should this happen, we can give you drugs to overcome it.

Dry mouth is other side effects which can be overcome by frequent drinks or artificial saliva.

Constipation is another side effect, which can be avoided if you eat a lot of vegetables and fruits, especially those with high fibres and even we can give you some laxatives.

Also this medication may cause *difficulty to pass water* and should this happen, try to go to toilet and turn on the tap, relax and you may pass water; but if it didn't work, you should come to hospital.

Other side effects are *sleepiness* (avoid driving) and *respiratory depression*, which occurs, only in high doses.

There is another entity, which is called *dependence* and this happens when large doses of this medication are used for a long time. But because we are going to start you on small doses that chance is very slim. Besides, we are unable to control your pain without this medication that is why it is very important to consider taking it."

"Is everything clear? Do you have any questions to ask?"

"Thank you very much for your co-operation."

CARCINOMA OF PROSTATE, OPTIONS OF PAIN RELIEF

Greet, introduce yourself and identify the patient.

"I need to have a few words with you about your condition. Is that OK?"

"As you know you have a growth in your prostate and this might cause you some pain.

Fortunately, we have a wide range of medications for pain relief. Paracetamol, in higher doses, may affect the liver."

NSAIDS - Aspirin and Indomethacin.

"They are also effective and given by mouth and should be taken with food to reduce their gastric irritation effect.

They might cause some tummy pain, blood in the motion or black-coloured motion. These medications can be combined with weak opioids as dextro-propoxyphene to become more effective.

Opioids as morphine, are very effective but have some side effects such as feeling sick, being sick, constipation, sleepiness and low mood.

However, we can deal with these side-effects by adjusting the medication dose or by giving laxatives and antiemetics.

Another option that we have for pain relief is to use radiotherapy, which is especially useful for bone pain. However, it may have some side effects as going frequently to toilet to pass water, feeling the urge to pass water suddenly, redness of skin and you need to come to hospital daily for 4–6 weeks to have the treatment.

Decreasing the male hormone, that is testosterone, is yet another method of pain relief and this can be done either by giving some medication or removing both testicles, but this may affect sexual performance."

"Is everything clear? Have you got any questions?"

"Thank you very much for your co-operation."

COLONOSCOPY

Greet, introduce yourself and identify the patient.

Ascertain how much does the patient know about the procedure?

"It is performed using IV sedation, which also has amnesic effect. Someone has to drive you back home."

Explain the procedure and its purpose to the patient
"The procedure is performed using colonoscope which is a flexible, thin tube as thin as a finger (1 cm) with a tiny camera attached to its end and passed through the back passage. The procedure is performed by an experienced doctor. It takes almost 20 minutes.

The very thought of someone putting a tube in back passage is not pleasant, but it is absolutely necessary as it is the only means by which you can find the exact nature of the problem.

The doctor is going to see inside your bowel and he may take a few pin-sized tissues from the lining of your bowel to examine them under the microscope to identify the nature of the problem."

Pre-procedure preparations

"We'll give you a medication (picolax) in the form of a powder to take it the day before the procedure with clear fluids only and you should not take anything else please."

Side effects

Discomfort during and after the procedure (cramping and bloating).

Bleeding from bowel lining (biopsy).

Drowsiness and short-term forgetfulness.

Tear in the wall of the bowel

A defunctioning colostomy may be required if there is:

- Peritoneal soilage.
- Infection.
- Intestinal obstruction.

Post-procedure observation

"You need to stay at hospital for 2 hours after the procedure to make sure that everything is fine and when you go home, please contact your doctor if you have tummy pain, bleeding, temperature or chills."

Ask about any concerns

"Here is the consent form. Can you read it and sign it please."

"Thank you very much for your co-operation."

LUMBAR PUNCTURE

Greet, introduce yourself and identify the patient.

Enquire if the patient knows about the procedure?

Explain the procedure and its details to him/her.

"We are going to withdraw tiny drops of fluid which is present in the backbone to reach a diagnosis."

Reassure by saying "The procedure is relatively simple and with experienced hands it takes only a few minutes. It is done by a well-trained staff."

Procedure

Positions: "During the procedure you are going to be placed in left lateral position with the backbone parallel and on the edge of the bed. Or, you may have to stand upright leaning over a support, such as the patients table covered with pillows.

In both the positions we adjust the height of the bed to allow comfort and ease during the procedure.

You will feel some pushing on the back and around the top of the hips as the landmarks are mapped out your skin is cleaned with an antiseptic which is cold and then the lower back is covered with surgical sheets.

You will feel some more pushing as the needle is inserted through the skin.

A small amount of fluid (3 ml) is then drained from your spine and this is sent to the laboratory to be looked at under the microscope.

You will be expected to lie flat for 6–8 hours after the procedure and you will be given analgesia and fluids."

Complications

Local pain at the puncture site and headache are the primary problems.

Ask for any concerns.

"Here is the consent form. Can you please read it, sign it and date it?"

"Thank you very much for your co-operation."

UNPROTECTED SEX, HIV

Greet, introduce, identify, acknowledge and ask for consent.

"I understand that you are worried because you had unprotected sex. I need to ask you a few questions and I can assure you that whatever you say to me will be strictly confidential. Is that alright?"

"Could you please tell me more about that?

When did you have sex?

With whom did you have sex?

How many times did you have sex with that person on the same day?

Did you penetrate her?

Did you use any condoms?

Did you notice anything in the lady? Any infection?

Have you got any discharge from penis/front passage?

Any itch, rash, sore, blisters or pain in your private areas?

Any pain or burning sensation while passing water?

Passing water more than usual with little quantity?

Pain during sex?

Any temperature?

Any joint pain?

I can assure you that the chance of getting HIV by a single act of unprotected sex is slim but we should not neglect it.

I can refer you to GUM clinic where you will have free check up and treatment and everything is kept strictly confidential.

You can have tests for HIV, hepatitis (HbsAg), swabs from any secretion or discharges from your private areas and other urine tests (for gonorrhoea and chlamydia) and blood tests (for syphilis).

HIV test results may be false negative due to window periods, so we have to repeat the test after 3, 6 and 8 months.

If the result is positive, it has to be confirmed by another test, which is called 'Western Blot test'.

It is very important to consider using barrier contraceptives as condoms until it is all clear and it would be advised to avoid having recreational drugs by needle exchanges."

"Any question?"

EPILEPSY (LIFESTYLE)

Epilepsy means that there is some abnormal electrical activity in her brain since the cause is not known she has nothing to blame herself for.

Introduction.

"I need to have a few words with you about minimal change you may need to do in your lifestyle."

General

Allow enough time for work, rest and different activities.

Eat regular meals (avoid prolonged period without food).

Have regular sleep (probability of fits).

Take sufficient medication with you when you go away from home.

It's a good idea to wear a Medic-Alert chain or bracelet to let people know about your condition.

At home

Living room: Stay away from fire.

Choose a soft carpet.

Fit safety glass in windows and doors.

TV at 8 feet, computer at 3 feet.

Kitchen: Don't cook on your own.

Microwaves are safer than cookers.

Turn the sauce pan handle towards the other side.

Carry the plates to the pan and not vice versa.

Bedroom: Use wide low-level bed.

Bathroom: Let people know, who know you, that you are having a shower. Having a shower is safer than bathing.

Don't lock the door.

Turn off the tap before you get in and it's better to keep the water shallow.

At work: Avoid operating heavy machinery or going up to high open spaces.

Driving: You will have to inform DVLA. You mustn't drive by law until you are 2 year fit-free when awake, or 3 year fit-free when sleeping.

Avoid heights

Sports: Carry on: jogging, tennis, basketball and swimming, but avoid dangerous sports such as horse riding, parachuting and paragliding because it's difficult for people to reach you when you need help.

Recreational drugs should be completely avoided, alcohol could be taken in moderation, you should *stop smoking*.

(*Alcohol*: 1 pint of beer, 2 glasses of wine or 2 measures of spirit.)

Pregnancy: Antiepileptics decrease the efficacy of OCP. You should use alternative methods like barrier method. Antiepileptics are teratogenic, no problem with pregnancy, but you should inform your obstetrician."

BRONCHOSCOPY AND BIOPSY

Greet, introduce yourself and identify the patient.

Enqyire how much does the patient know about the procedure?

Explain the procedure and its purpose to the patient.

“The bronchoscope is a flexible, thin tube which is as thin as a finger with a tiny camera attached to its end and inserted down into the windpipe. The instrument is thin enough to allow breathing.”

“Bronchoscopy is performed by an experienced doctor and they are going to numb your airways by a spray. The anaesthetist will talk to you later about that.

The procedure takes about 20 minutes.

The doctor is going to look at your airways and s/he may take tiny pieces of tissue from your airways just to examine them under microscope to identify the nature of the problem

You can go home on the same day but you should not drive because the anaesthesia makes you drowsy.”

Complications

“Sore throat.

Some chest discomfort.

Post-procedure drowsiness.

Bleeding into the lungs.

Perforation of the windpipe and smaller airways causing collection of air in your chest wall or inside your lungs (pneumo-mediustinum, pneumo-thorax and surgical emphysema), in which case there might be the need for insertion of a chest drain tube.

Chest infection, if any, will be treated by antibiotics.

"Here is the consent form, can you please read it, sign it and date it?"

"Thank you very much for your co-operation."

READERS' NOTES

READERS' NOTES

READERS' NOTES

READERS' NOTES

READERS' NOTES

READERS' NOTES